The ULTIMATE HOLISTIC ESSENTIALS

2 IN 1

A Complete Wellness and Fitness Collection with Mindfulness and Healthy Diet for Everyday Living

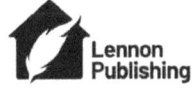

Copyright © 2025 by Lennon Publishing

All rights reserved.

No portion of this book may be reproduced in any form without written permission from the publisher or author, except as permitted by U.S. copyright law.

This publication is designed to provide accurate and authoritative information in regard to the subject matter covered. It is sold with the understanding that neither the author nor the publisher is engaged in rendering legal, investment, accounting or other professional services. While the publisher and author have used their best efforts in preparing this book, they make no representations or warranties with respect to the accuracy or completeness of the contents of this book and specifically disclaim any implied warranties of merchantability or fitness for a particular purpose. No warranty may be created or extended by sales representatives or written sales materials. The advice and strategies contained herein may not be suitable for your situation. You should consult with a professional when appropriate. Neither the publisher nor the author shall be liable for any loss of profit or any other commercial damages, including but not limited to special, incidental, consequential, personal, or other damages.

Portions previously published in 2025 as second editions of *Holistic Living for Wellness: Your Guide to Spiritual Growth, Healthy Diet, and a Fitness Plan Even If Life Gets Busy* and *Holistic Living for Fitness: A Mindful Approach to Workouts, Meal Planning, and Lasting Weight Loss in a Hectic World* and

First Edition 2025

Contents

Note To The Reader   X

Holistic Living for Wellness: Your Guide to Spiritual Growth, Healthy Diet, and a Fitness Plan Even If Life Gets Busy

  Contents   3

  1. Foundations of Holistic Wellness   4

    Understanding Holistic Health: More Than Just the Body

    The Psychology of Self-Care: Why Your Mind Matters

    Emotional Wellness: Recognizing and Managing Emotions

    Integrating Mindfulness into Everyday Life

    The Science of Stress and its Holistic Counteractions

    Setting Realistic Wellness Goals That Resonate with Your Lifestyle

    Chapter 1 Wellness Plan: Introduction to Holistic Wellness

  2. Nutrition for the Mind and Body   22

    Balanced Diets for Busy Professionals: Quick and Nutritious Choices
    Superfoods and Their Role in Mental Clarity
    Managing Dietary Needs Without Stress
    The Impact of Hydration on Physical and Mental Performance
    Planning Meals for Energy and Focus
    Integrating Nutritional Strategies with Family Dining
    Chapter 2 Wellness Plan: Nutrition for the Mind and Body

3. Physical Fitness in a Busy World   42
    Designing a Flexible Fitness Routine
    High-Intensity Interval Training (HIIT) for Time-Savers
    The Role of Walking: Underrated Exercises
    The Importance of Rest and Recovery
    Chapter 3 Wellness Plan: Physical Fitness in a Busy World

4. Mental, Emotional, and Spiritual Health Nourishment   64
    Practical Mindfulness Exercises for Anxiety
    Cognitive Behavioral Techniques Without the Jargon
    Building Resilience Against Daily Stressors
    Managing Social Anxiety Through Small Steps
    Enhancing Sleep Quality for Emotional Well-being

Tech Tools That Aid Mental Wellness
Art and Music Therapy: Creative Outlets for Stress Relief
Chapter 4 Wellness Plan: Emotional and Mental Wellness

5. Spiritual Growth and Personal Faith …… 89
   Daily Practices for Spiritual Growth
   Meditation and Its Varieties: Finding What Fits
   The Role of Nature in Spiritual Wellness
   Creating a Personal Ritual for Spiritual Health
   Faith Across Cultures: Universal Wellness Lessons
   The Benefits of Spiritual Retreats in Everyday Settings
   Chapter 5 Wellness Plan: Spiritual Growth and Personal Faith

6. Sustainable Living and Wellness …… 110
   Eco-Friendly Choices That Enhance Personal Health
   Reducing Your Carbon Footprint with Smarter Food Choices
   Sustainable Fitness: Environmentally Conscious Exercise
   Household Toxins and Natural Alternatives
   The Wellness Benefits of Minimalism
   Community Gardening and Local Food Sources
   Chapter 6 Wellness Plan: Sustainable Living and Wellness

7. Social Wellness and Community Building   133
   Building Supportive Relationships
   Communicating Needs and Boundaries
   Volunteering: The Health Benefits of Giving Back
   Group Fitness and Social Bonds
   Online Communities for Holistic Health Support
   Wellness Workshops and Local Events
   Chapter 7 Wellness Plan: Social Wellness and Community Building

8. Adapting Wellness Into Your Unique Lifestyle   155
   Tailoring Wellness Practices for Different Life Stages
   Overcoming the Guilt of Self-Care
   Integrating Wellness into the Workday
   The Role of Personal Development in Wellness
   Keeping Wellness Engaging and New
   Reviewing and Renewing Your Wellness Goals Annually
   Chapter 8 Wellness Plan: Adapting Wellness Into Your Unique Lifestyle

9. Bonus Chapter: Ask the Wellness Coach   179

10. Conclusion   186

References   190

Holistic Living for Fitness : A Mindful Approach to Workouts, Meal Planning, and Lasting Weight Loss in a Hectic World

Contents   197

Introduction   198

1. Embracing the Mind-Body Connection   201
   Understanding Holistic Fitness
   The Science of Mindfulness in Exercise
   Cultivating Awareness in Movement
   Breathing Techniques for Mental Clarity
   Body Scanning for Stress Reduction
   Integrating Mindfulness into Daily Routines

2. Mindful Nutrition Essentials   225
   Building a Balanced Plate with Intention
   Recognizing Hunger and Fullness Cues
   Savoring Food: Techniques for Slowing Down
   Emotional Eating: Identifying and Overcoming Triggers
   Sustainable Meal Planning and Prep

3. Personalized Fitness for Every Lifestyle   247
   Time-Efficient Workouts for Busy Schedules
   Functional Fitness for Everyday Life
   Low-Impact Exercises for All Ages
   Incorporating Yoga and Stretching for Flexibility
   Strength Training for Beginners

4. Creating Lasting Habits   269
   Habit Stacking for Seamless Integration
   Overcoming Barriers to Change
   Setting Realistic and Achievable Goals
   Maintaining Motivation Through Accountability
   Tracking Progress and Celebrating Milestones

5. Mindful Living and Stress Management — 287
    Mindfulness Techniques for Stress Relief
    The Power of Meditation in Daily Life
    Prioritizing Sleep for Optimal Health
    Digital Detox: Reclaiming Your Mind for Mindfulness
    The Impact of Digital Overload
    The Benefits of a Digital Detox
    Practical Steps for a Digital Detox
    Reclaiming Balance and Presence
    Cultivating a Positive Mindset

6. Ethical and Environmental Considerations — 303
    Interactive Journal: Ethical Shopping Checklist
    Navigating Plant-Based Nutrition
    Balancing Ethical Eating with Personal Health
    Reducing Food Waste: Practical Tips
    Sustainable Sourcing: Making Informed Choices
    The Environmental Impact of Dietary Choices

7. Interactive Journaling for Self-Discovery — 321
    Journaling Prompts for Mindful Eating
    Tracking Emotional Well-Being
    Visualizing Your Health Goals
    Gratitude Practices for Positivity
    Creating a Personalized Wellness Journal

8. Enhancing Your Wellness Journey with Technology — 340
    Interactive Journal: Fitness App Evaluation Checklist

      Digital Tools for Tracking Nutrition
      Online Communities for Support and Motivation
      Virtual Workouts: Finding What Works for You
      Mindfulness Apps to Enhance Meditation
      Balancing Screen Time with Mindful Living

9. Conclusion   359

Extended Edition: Travel-Friendly Workouts   362
   Sample Travel Day Plan

Bonus Chapter: Fitness Myths Debunked   369
Separating Fact from Fiction

References   378

Note To The Reader

We're thrilled to present the Holistic Living Essentials Collection, bringing together the Second Editions of Holistic Living for Wellness and Holistic Living for Fitness in one complete guide.

These updated editions reflect everything our readers loved most, deeper spiritual reflections, refreshed meal plans, and the new Ask the Wellness Coach Q&A in Wellness, alongside the Travel-Friendly Workouts and extended routines in Fitness.

This collection was created for readers who want to explore both mindfulness and movement as one continuous journey. Whether you begin with stillness or strength, you'll find guidance designed to meet you where you are, with practical tools to support balance in everyday life. Dive in at your own pace, return to sections that speak to you, and let these two guides work together toward one goal: a more grounded, energized, and intentional you.

First Edition, 2025

HOLISTIC LIVING *for* WELLNESS

Your Guide to Spiritual Growth, Healthy Diet, and a Fitness Plan Even If Life Gets Busy

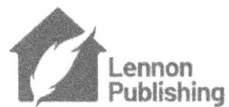

Contents

1. Foundations of Holistic Wellness — 4
2. Nutrition for the Mind and Body — 22
3. Physical Fitness in a Busy World — 42
4. Mental, Emotional, and Spiritual Health Nourishment — 64
5. Spiritual Growth and Personal Faith — 89
6. Sustainable Living and Wellness — 110
7. Social Wellness and Community Building — 133
8. Adapting Wellness Into Your Unique Lifestyle — 155
9. Bonus Chapter: Ask the Wellness Coach — 179
10. Conclusion — 186

References — 190

Chapter 1

Foundations of Holistic Wellness

In the hustle of our daily routines, where deadlines, family obligations, and personal projects collide, the quest for health often becomes a footnote—a wishful note scribbled on the back pages of our minds. Yet, what if I told you that embracing a holistic approach to wellness could transform that footnote into the headline of your life's story, not just enhancing your longevity but enriching the quality of every moment? This chapter is dedicated to unfolding the layers of holistic wellness, a concept that integrates your physical, mental, emotional, and spiritual well-being, allowing you to thrive in a world that doesn't pause.

Understanding Holistic Health: More Than Just the Body

Holistic health is an invitation to explore wellness beyond the conventional scope. It's not merely about preventing or treating diseases; it's about nurturing a harmonious balance that enriches your life. This approach recognizes you as a complete entity, intertwining your physical, mental, emotional, and spiritual health. Take, for instance, how emerging research continues to reveal the profound connection between gut health and mental well-being. It's fascinating to discover that the simple act of nurturing your gut flora with a diet rich in fibers and probiotics can elevate your mood and cognitive function, illustrating a perfect example of how physical health impacts mental clarity.

Throughout history, holistic health practices have been a fundamental part of countless cultures worldwide. From the use of Ayurveda in India and traditional Chinese medicine in Asia to herbalism in indigenous cultures, these practices, though diverse in application, share a common principle: the belief in treating the individual as an interconnected whole rather than a series of parts. Over centuries, these ancient wisdoms have not only persisted but have also evolved, integrating seamlessly with modern medical practices to offer us a comprehensive view of health and wellness.

Contrasting sharply with conventional Western medicine, holistic health does not focus solely on symptoms but seeks to address the root causes of illness. Where traditional medicine might prescribe medication to relieve symptoms, a holistic approach considers the broader spectrum of an individual's lifestyle, environment, and emotional health. This might mean recommending changes to diet, exercise, social habits, and stress management as part of the treatment plan. It's a form of medicine that's as preventative as it is curative, emphasizing natural remedies and lifestyle changes over pharmaceutical solutions whenever possible.

Today, the acceptance of holistic health practices has seen a remarkable surge in modern healthcare settings. More physicians than ever before are prescribing integrative therapies like acupuncture, yoga, and meditation alongside conventional medical treatments. This shift reflects a growing recognition within the healthcare community of the benefits these ancient practices bring to modern medicine. For instance, hospitals incorporating stress-reduction programs based on mindfulness techniques have reported improvements in patient recovery rates and reductions in hospital stays.

As holistic health continues to weave its way into the fabric of modern medicine, it invites us to rethink our approach to health and wellness. It encourages us to consider not just the physical symptoms but the complex interplay of all aspects of our being. By doing so, it offers a more sustainable, empowering, and compassionate approach to healthcare, one that respects both the science of medicine and the art of healing.

The Psychology of Self-Care: Why Your Mind Matters

Understanding the role of mental health in overall well-being is pivotal. In our bustling daily lives, the mind often bears the brunt of our stress, juggling deadlines, relationships, and our aspirations. Research continually underscores the profound impact that stress has on physical health, ranging from weakened immune systems to increased risk of chronic diseases like hypertension and diabetes. The symbiotic relationship between mind and body is crucial for holistic wellness, emphasizing the importance of nurturing both mental and physical health for overall well-being. This intricate interplay highlights why mental health is not just a side note in the narrative of wellness but a central theme.

Self-care, often misconstrued as a luxury or indulgence, is a fundamental practice for mental health. Engaging in self-care activities like journaling offers a reflective pause from the daily grind, providing a space to process thoughts and emotions, leading to greater self-awareness and a reduced sense of overwhelm. Meditation, another cornerstone of self-care, allows for a mental breather, a moment to detach from the chaos of life and return with a calmer, more focused mind. Socializing, too, plays a critical role. It strengthens connections, provides emotional support, and often, a fresh perspective on personal challenges. The psychological benefits of these activities are profound—they not only enhance mood and energy levels but also fortify cognitive functions, making them essential tools in your wellness arsenal.

However, the path to regular self-care is often obstructed by psychological barriers. Guilt is a significant hurdle, with many perceiving self-care as selfish or unwarranted, especially when other responsibilities demand their attention. This guilt intensifies in a society that often glorifies relentless work and perpetual activity, neglecting the importance of rest and recovery. Overcoming these barriers begins with redefining self-care as a necessary practice that enhances our capacity to engage with life. By shifting the narrative to view self-care as an act of kindness to oneself, and by extension to those we interact with, it becomes easier to prioritize these practices without the accompanying guilt.

Cultivating resilience, essential for overcoming life's obstacles, is deeply intertwined with mindful self-care. It's about shaping a mindset that interprets obstacles as avenues for growth and perceives errors as essential steps in the learning journey. Such an outlook is fostered through mindfulness practices that emphasize the importance of being present and responding thoughtfully to situations instead of reacting impulsively. Consider resilience as a muscle that gains strength through regular exercise; similarly, by consistently practicing self-care strategies such as setting achievable goals, seeking emotional support when necessary, and maintaining an optimistic attitude, you enhance your ability to handle stress and recover from difficulties more efficiently.

As we explore these facets of mental wellness, it becomes clear that the mind is not just a vessel to be filled, but a complex system to be nurtured and cared for. In the subsequent sections, we delve into the practical applications of these concepts, ensuring that you are equipped not only with the knowledge but also the tools to foster a resilient, healthy mind.

Emotional Wellness: Recognizing and Managing Emotions

At the core of holistic health, emotional wellness plays a pivotal role, yet it frequently slips under the radar amid our bustling lives. It's about acknowledging and valuing our emotions as crucial indicators that shed light on our overall health and shape how we interact with the world. Far from mere sentiments, emotions serve as essential alerts, signaling the state of our internal and external realms. They act as barometers for assessing the fulfillment of our needs and our connection to our surroundings. For instance, a continuous sense of sadness may suggest a longing for deeper relationships or more purposeful activities, whereas ongoing annoyance might point to overstretched limits, highlighting the need for firmer boundaries or the delegation of tasks.

This understanding leads us into the realm of emotional intelligence, a skill set that includes self-awareness, empathy, self-regulation, motivation, and social skills. Emotional intelligence profoundly impacts both personal and professional relationships, influencing how we communicate, resolve conflicts, and lead others. Self-awareness allows us to recognize our emotional triggers and understand their origins, which is the first step in managing them effectively. Empathy extends this awareness to others, enabling us to perceive and react to the emotions of those around us, thus fostering stronger and more harmonious relationships.

Managing our emotions, particularly intense ones such as anger or sadness requires practical strategies that can be seamlessly integrated into everyday life. Breathing exercises, for instance, are a powerful tool for regulating emotional responses. The simple act of taking deep, controlled breaths can activate the body's relaxation response, helping to calm the mind and reduce the intensity of emotional reactions. Mindfulness practices also play a crucial role in emotional regulation. By bringing our attention to the present moment and observing our thoughts and feelings without judgment, we can gain critical insights into the patterns of our emotional responses and develop greater mastery over them.

Cognitive reframing is another valuable technique in the emotional wellness toolkit. This strategy involves changing our perspective on a situation to alter its emotional impact. For example, viewing a stressful work project as an opportunity to develop new skills rather than a burden can significantly reduce feelings of anxiety and increase motivation. Real-life scenarios demonstrate the effectiveness of these techniques. Consider a professional faced with a daunting deadline. By practicing mindfulness, the individual can maintain focus and reduce panic, and by using cognitive reframing, they can transform anxiety into a driving force that enhances performance rather than a paralyzing fear.

These case studies not only highlight the practical applications of emotional wellness strategies but also underscore the transformative impact they can have on life outcomes and relationships. A person who masters emotional self-regulation is better equipped to handle interpersonal challenges, lead with confidence, and maintain a positive outlook in the face of adversity. This mastery does not come overnight but through consistent practice and a commitment to self-growth. By integrating these practices into our daily routines, we empower ourselves to lead more balanced, fulfilling lives, where emotions are not obstacles but valuable guides that lead us toward greater well-being.

Integrating Mindfulness into Everyday Life

Mindfulness, a term that's seen a surge in popularity but is often surrounded by misconceptions, is essentially about being fully present and engaged at the moment, aware of your thoughts and feelings without distraction or judgment. This practice, rooted deeply in Buddhist meditation, has been scientifically shown to modify the structures and functions of the brain, leading to improved mental clarity and reduced stress levels. Studies, like those published in the *Journal of Management*, indicate that mindfulness meditation can significantly decrease stress and enhance cognitive functions such as concentration, memory, and learning agility. Imagine the benefits of being less reactive to stressors at work or more attentive during conversations with loved ones. This isn't just about reducing stress; it's about enhancing the quality of every moment of your day.

Integrating mindfulness into daily activities can start with something as simple as mindful eating. This involves paying full attention to the experience of eating—observing the colors, smells, textures, and flavors of your food, and noticing the responses it evokes within your body. This practice not only enhances your enjoyment of meals but can also help regulate appetite and improve digestion. For instance, by eating mindfully, you might notice when you are full, reducing the likelihood of overeating. Similarly, mindful walking—where you focus intently on the movement of your body and the sensation of your feet touching the ground—can transform a routine walk to the subway into a revitalizing break from the mental chatter of your day.

Another practical way to incorporate mindfulness is during daily routines like showering or commuting. While showering, for instance, you can focus on the sensation of water on your skin, the sound of the water droplets, and the scent of your soap, turning a mundane activity into a refreshing ritual that clears your mind. If you commute, try turning off the car radio for a few minutes or put away your phone if you're on public transport. Use this time to breathe deeply and observe your surroundings, noting anything you can see, hear, or feel. This isn't just about 'killing time' but making the most of these moments to rejuvenate your mind.

In the workplace, mindfulness has proven its worth beyond just being a personal wellness tool; it enhances productivity and creativity. Incorporating mindfulness techniques like scheduled breathing breaks or a few minutes of guided meditation can help manage work-related stress, fostering a calmer mind that's better equipped to tackle complex tasks and brainstorm creative solutions. Research from the *Mindfulness Journal* suggests that mindfulness practices can reduce mental fatigue and burnout caused by multitasking and constant digital connectivity, common challenges in today's workplace settings.

By embedding mindfulness into the fabric of our daily lives, we not only improve our well-being but also bring greater attentiveness and care into our interactions with others. Whether it's through a deeper engagement with our work, more meaningful conversations with family, or simply enjoying a meal without the distraction of our screens, mindfulness offers a way to live richer, more fulfilled lives. The beauty of mindfulness lies in its simplicity and accessibility; it doesn't require special equipment or unusual skills, just a commitment to paying attention to the here and now. By embracing these practices, you can start to see significant changes, not just in your mental health, but in all aspects of your life, reinforcing the interconnectedness of your experiences and your wellness.

The Science of Stress and its Holistic Counteractions

Stress, a constant companion in both our professional and personal realms, has become a staple of modern life. At the heart of stress lies the body's ancient fight-or-flight mechanism, an instinctual response that unleashes a surge of hormones like cortisol and adrenaline to prepare us for immediate action. While this mechanism was crucial for survival in natural environments, it's less beneficial amidst the non-stop demands of today's world, such as endless emails and consecutive meetings. The very hormones that equip our forebears to evade predators persist in our bodies, leading to physical manifestations such as a faster heartbeat, elevated blood pressure, and a compromised immune system. This persistent state of alert not only depletes our bodily systems but also impacts our overall health, paving the way for a spectrum of issues including digestive disturbances and cardiovascular diseases.

Turning to holistic stress management, practices such as yoga and tai chi offer more than just a moment of calm. These ancient techniques stand out for their dual ability to soothe the mind and fortify the body. Yoga, with its series of postures and controlled breathing exercises, helps in reducing tension and enhancing blood circulation, which in turn lowers blood pressure and boosts mood. Similarly, tai chi, often described as meditation in motion, promotes serenity through gentle movements, reducing the body's stress responses and improving physical balance and stamina. Beyond these, herbal supplements like ashwagandha and lavender are lauded for their natural soothing properties that can help stabilize the body's cortisol levels, thus supporting the body's natural resilience against stress.

The fabric of community and social connections also plays a pivotal role in buffering against stress. Sociological studies have consistently shown that strong social networks enhance an individual's ability to manage stress and recover from illness more quickly. This support system can be as simple as having someone to talk through daily frustrations with or as involved as community groups that provide social interaction and collective problem-solving. Engaging with others can mitigate feelings of isolation and helplessness that often accompany high stress, providing not just emotional comfort but also practical assistance and advice. For instance, consider how a support group for new parents can alleviate the stress of child-rearing by offering a platform to share experiences, advice, and encouragement, reinforcing not only individual coping capacity but also fostering collective resilience.

However, the stakes of ignoring stress management are high. Chronic stress, if left unchecked, can lead to serious health issues such as cardiovascular diseases and mental disorders like depression and anxiety. These conditions not only diminish the quality of life but also place a burden on healthcare systems. Through holistic practices, which advocate for a preventative approach, the risks associated with prolonged stress can be significantly mitigated. Embracing a lifestyle that incorporates stress-management techniques, community support, and natural remedies not only enhances your immediate well-being but also sets the foundation for a healthier, more vibrant life.

Setting Realistic Wellness Goals That Resonate with Your Lifestyle

Embarking on a wellness journey that aligns with your life circumstances involves more than just temporary changes; it's about implementing changes that endure. Developing a personal wellness plan that addresses your physical, mental, emotional, and spiritual well-being is comparable to charting a map toward your optimal self. The challenge lies not only in plotting this course but also in crafting it to be practical and achievable within the complexities of your daily life.

Crafting a wellness plan is akin to nurturing a garden, requiring it to be customized to fit the unique dynamics of your life, whether that's the pace of your career or the demands of family life. Start by examining every aspect of your health. Set goals to increase physical activity or improve your diet, aim for better stress management and deepen connections with loved ones for mental and emotional well-being. For spiritual health, dedicate time to meditation or connecting with nature. The beauty of a holistic approach lies in understanding how improvements in one area can positively impact others. For instance, regular physical activity not only boosts heart health but also enhances mood and vitality through endorphin release, encouraging more social and spiritual engagement.

Setting goals is a craft in itself. They should be SMART—Specific, Measurable, Achievable, Relevant, and Time-bound. Specific goals dispel ambiguity, guiding you toward success with clarity. Measurable objectives enable progress tracking, offering a sense of accomplishment as you achieve milestones. Goals should be Achievable to avoid discouragement and sufficiently challenging to stimulate growth. They must also be Relevant to your broader life ambitions and Time-bound, with a realistic deadline for completion. For instance, instead of a vague aim to "eat healthier," a SMART goal could be "to incorporate two servings of vegetables into my dinner five nights a week for the next month." This approach not only integrates the goal into your routine but also ensures it's practical and measurable.

Life, however, is not static. It throws curveballs like a new job across the country, the birth of a child, or unexpected personal challenges. These changes can derail even the most well-thought-out wellness plan. The key is adaptability. When major life changes occur, take them as opportunities to reassess and adjust your goals. Perhaps after moving to a new city, your goal to jog in the local park every morning becomes impractical due to a longer commute. You might switch to weekend hikes or find a closer gym. The ability to pivot and reshape your wellness strategies around new circumstances is crucial. It ensures that your approach to health and wellness grows with you, reflecting your current realities rather than remaining a relic of your past.

Continuous learning and adaptation are key to evolving your wellness journey. As health trends shift and personal needs change, especially with aging, it's crucial to stay updated on wellness practices. This may involve transitioning from high-intensity workouts to gentler activities like yoga or incorporating mindfulness to ease career stress. Connecting with a supportive community, be it through local classes, online forums, or friend groups, enriches this journey with shared insights and encouragement. Ultimately, the aim is to develop a flexible wellness plan that fits your current lifestyle and future goals. Prioritizing health with this adaptable strategy enables you to face life's challenges head-on. A well-integrated wellness approach fosters habits that boost happiness and fulfillment.

> *"Holistic wellness begins with the foundation of nurturing the mind, body, and spirit, creating a balanced life that thrives on harmony and well-being."*

Chapter 1 Wellness Plan: Introduction to Holistic Wellness

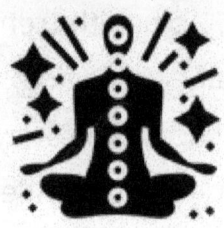

Activity: Setting Your Wellness Goals

Identify Your Goals

List three specific wellness goals you want to achieve (e.g., improve sleep quality, increase physical activity, reduce stress).

Daily Habits

Write down one daily habit you can adopt for each goal (e.g., go to bed at the same time every night, take a 20-minute walk, practice deep breathing).

Weekly Check-In

Schedule a time at the end of each week to reflect on your progress. Note any challenges and adjust your habits as needed.

Reflection Questions:

★ *What motivated you to choose these goals?*

★ *How do you feel when you make progress toward these goals?*

Meditation: Visualization (5 minutes)
　★ *Sit comfortably and close your eyes.*
　★ *Take a few deep breaths and relax your body.*
　★*Visualize yourself achieving one of your wellness goals.*
　★*Imagine the positive impact it has on your life and how you feel achieving it.*

Suggested Music:
　★ **Ambient Music:** *Brian Eno's "Music for Airports"*
　★ **Instrumental Guitar:** *Andy McKee's "Art of Motion"*

By regularly reflecting on your goals and progress, you can stay motivated and make meaningful strides toward holistic wellness. Use the visualization meditation to strengthen your commitment and envision the positive changes in your life.

Chapter 2

Nutrition for the Mind and Body

Imagine this: it's late afternoon, you're just finishing a hectic workday, and your energy levels are hitting a new low. We've all been there, right? Now, amid the chaos, reaching for that candy bar feels like a quick fix. But what if your desk drawer was stocked with nutrient-packed snacks that not only satisfy your hunger but also boost your energy and focus? This chapter is dedicated to transforming how you think about food, making nutrition an integral and effortless part of your busy lifestyle. Let's explore how a balanced diet can be your secret weapon for maintaining high energy, sharp focus, and overall well-being—even on your busiest days.

Balanced Diets for Busy Professionals: Quick and Nutritious Choices

The foundation of maintaining energy and focus throughout a demanding day lies in the power of balanced nutrition. But let's be real: when your schedule is packed, spending hours preparing complex meals isn't just impractical; it's nearly impossible. That's where the magic of quick-prep, nutritious foods comes into play. Foods like Greek yogurt with a handful of nuts, smoothies packed with fruits and vegetables, or whole-grain wraps filled with lean protein such as turkey or hummus are not only easy to prepare but are also incredibly nutrient-dense. These options provide a balanced mix of proteins, fats, and carbohydrates, which are essential for sustaining energy. For instance, starting your day with a smoothie that includes spinach, a banana, and a scoop of protein powder can keep you satiated and sharp for hours.

Now, let's talk about meal prepping, a strategy that can revolutionize your eating habits without burdening your schedule. The concept is simple: dedicate a few hours over the weekend to prepare large batches of meals that can be easily stored and quickly served throughout the week. Think of cooking a large tray of roasted vegetables, grilling several chicken breasts, or preparing a big pot of quinoa. These can then be mixed and matched to create different meals throughout the week, saving you a significant amount of time and decision-making each day. Moreover, embracing the use of healthy, ready-made options like pre-cut vegetables or canned beans can further streamline your meal preparation process, ensuring you always have the building blocks of a healthy meal at hand, even when time is not on your side.

Balancing macronutrients is another key aspect of a nutritionally sound diet, especially important when your days demand a lot from you. Proteins, fats, and carbohydrates play distinct and vital roles in your body. Proteins are essential for building and repairing tissues; fats provide a long-lasting source of energy and aid in nutrient absorption; carbohydrates, particularly complex ones like those found in whole grains, are your body's main energy source. Ensuring that each meal includes a balanced proportion of these macronutrients can help maintain your energy levels consistently throughout the day. For example, a lunch that includes a grilled chicken salad with mixed greens (proteins and fats from chicken and dressing), a whole-grain roll (carbohydrates), and some avocado slices (healthy fats) is balanced and will keep you full and focused well into the afternoon.

Lastly, let's not forget about the importance of snacks. Healthy snacks play a crucial role in bridging meals and keeping hunger at bay, which helps in maintaining focus and preventing overeating at meal times. Portable, easy-to-carry snacks such as almonds, carrots with hummus, or an apple with peanut butter provide a quick energy boost and essential nutrients without the added sugars and unhealthy fats found in typical vending machine fare. Keeping these healthy snacks within easy reach throughout your day ensures that you're never too far from a nutritious energy boost, helping you manage your hunger and maintain your focus until your next meal.

By integrating these straightforward and practical nutritional strategies into your daily routine, you can ensure that even on the busiest days, your body and mind are well-nourished, keeping you energized and focused from morning until night. Whether it's choosing the right kinds of foods, prepping meals in advance, balancing your intake of macronutrients, or snacking smartly, these habits can transform your approach to daily nutrition, making a balanced diet an achievable and essential part of your high-performance lifestyle.

Superfoods and Their Role in Mental Clarity

The term "superfood" has become a buzzword in the wellness community, often evoking images of exotic berries and rare seeds. But what exactly qualifies a food as a "superfood"? Essentially, superfoods are nutrient powerhouses that pack large doses of antioxidants, vitamins, and minerals. They offer more bang for your nutritional buck, providing enhanced benefits that can support overall health, including brain function. For instance, consider foods like blueberries, known for their high levels of flavonoids which have been shown to improve memory and cognitive function. Then there's salmon, rich in omega-3 fatty acids, crucial for brain health and maintaining sharp cognitive abilities as we age.

The nutritional content of these superfoods is what sets them apart. Take dark leafy greens such as spinach and kale, which are loaded with vitamins A, C, E, and K, along with fiber, iron, magnesium, potassium, and calcium. These nutrients contribute not only to physical health but also support brain function by enhancing blood flow and reducing inflammatory processes within the brain, which can cloud mental clarity. Similarly, nuts and seeds like walnuts and flaxseeds offer omega-3 fatty acids and antioxidants that combat oxidative stress and inflammation in the brain, factors that can affect focus and clarity.

Incorporating these nutrient-dense foods into your daily meals doesn't require a complete overhaul of your diet or advanced culinary skills. Start simple by adding a handful of spinach to your morning smoothie or topping your yogurt with a mix of berries and seeds for an afternoon snack. Swap out your usual side of fries for a vibrant salad packed with mixed greens, avocado, nuts, and a sprinkle of chia seeds to not only satisfy your hunger but also feed your brain. These small, manageable adjustments can make a significant impact on your mental clarity and overall health.

However, it's essential to approach the superfood trend with a balanced perspective. While these foods are indeed beneficial, they are not cure-alls and should be part of a varied and balanced diet. Myths abound, suggesting that superfoods can single-handedly prevent diseases or offer miraculous health benefits. It's crucial to debunk these myths and recognize that while superfoods are helpful, they are most effective when consumed as part of a broader healthy lifestyle that includes regular physical activity and adequate hydration. No single food holds the key to good health, but a smart combination of these nutrient-rich foods can certainly contribute to maintaining a sharp and focused mind amidst the demands of your busy life.

Managing Dietary Needs Without Stress

Navigating the world of nutrition can often feel like trying to solve a complex puzzle, especially when you factor in individual dietary needs and restrictions. Whether these are due to health conditions, allergies, or personal wellness goals, understanding and managing these requirements shouldn't add extra stress to your already busy life. Let's walk through how you can identify your specific dietary needs and create a plan that flexibly fits into your lifestyle, ensuring that you can enjoy meals without worry, even in social settings.

Identifying your unique dietary needs is the first step toward a more personalized and effective nutrition plan. Start by considering any known health conditions or allergies that directly impact your diet. Consulting with a healthcare provider or a dietitian can provide a solid foundation of what foods to embrace or avoid. For instance, if you have diabetes, understanding the types of foods that influence blood sugar levels is crucial. Beyond medical advice, paying attention to how your body reacts to different foods can also guide your choices. Perhaps you notice that dairy products make you feel sluggish or bloated, suggesting a possible lactose sensitivity. Keeping a food diary can be an insightful tool in this journey, helping you track your food intake and your body's reactions, simplifying the identification of foods that support or hinder your well-being.

Once you've pinned down your dietary needs, the next challenge is crafting a diet plan that is both flexible and forgiving, accommodating the unexpected twists of daily life. The goal here is to create a framework that allows for adjustments without compromising nutritional balance or adding to your stress levels. Start by building a list of 'safe' foods that you know are good for you and that you enjoy eating. From this list, you can create a variety of mix-and-match meal options that can be quickly adapted based on your daily schedule and availability of ingredients. For example, if you're avoiding gluten, stocking up on gluten-free grains like quinoa and rice allows you to rotate your staples without mealtime becoming monotonous. Additionally, embracing the practice of batch cooking once or twice a week can ensure that you always have a base of healthy meals ready to go, which you can then tweak with different spices or fresh ingredients for variety.

In today's tech-driven world, numerous apps and resources can significantly simplify the task of tracking dietary intake and managing nutritional goals. Apps like MyFitnessPal or Yazio offer platforms where you can log daily meals and monitor your intake of macros and micronutrients, ensuring you stay on track with your dietary needs. These tools often come with customizable options where you can set reminders for meal times, water intake, and even grocery shopping lists that align with your dietary plans. This digital support not only aids in maintaining a consistent diet but also alleviates the mental load of having to remember every detail, allowing you to focus more on enjoying your food and less on managing it.

Handling dietary restrictions in social settings is often a concern for many, but it doesn't have to be a source of anxiety. When dining out, reviewing menus online beforehand or calling the restaurant to discuss your dietary needs can help ensure that there are suitable options for you, preventing any uncomfortable situations at the table. When attending social gatherings, offering to bring a dish that meets your dietary requirements can be a great way to participate without feeling restricted. It also introduces others to your type of diet, which can be a wonderful opportunity for sharing lifestyle choices and recipes. Communicating openly with friends and family about your dietary needs not only helps in managing social dining occasions but also builds understanding and support within your social circles, making these interactions more enjoyable and less stressful.

By taking these thoughtful steps, you can navigate your dietary needs with confidence and ease. From understanding what your body needs, crafting a flexible eating plan, leveraging digital tools for meal management, to navigating social meals without stress, each strategy is designed to support your dietary journey, making it a seamless part of your life rather than a constant challenge. This way, you can focus more on the joys of eating and less on the worries of what's on your plate.

The Impact of Hydration on Physical and Mental Performance

Fueling our bodies and minds for peak performance extends beyond nutrition and exercise; hydration plays a pivotal role, yet it's often overlooked. Drinking sufficient water impacts everything from our stamina to mental sharpness. It's essential for the optimal function of every cell, organ, and tissue. Water not only lubricates our joints and regulates body temperature but also ensures the delivery of vital nutrients throughout our body. Crucially, it supports brain functions, powering thought and memory processes. Achieving proper hydration means our brain can function efficiently, enhancing clarity, speed, and efficiency.

Grasping the science behind hydration reveals its profound effects on both body and mind, fundamentally altering how we view this everyday act. Hydration directly influences brain function and size; even slight dehydration can diminish cognitive abilities, complicate tasks and decision-making, and impair memory functions. A study in the Journal of Nutrition underscored that dehydration might result in attention deficits, slowed motor responses, and a heightened sense of difficulty in tasks.

Recognizing the importance of hydration, it's essential to personalize your daily water intake. Factors such as activity level, health status, and climate play a crucial role in determining your needs. Guidelines suggest about 3.7 liters for men and 2.7 liters for women as a baseline, inclusive of all fluids and food sources. However, these figures should be adjusted based on your physical activity and the environment you're in. It's important to attune to your body's signals, as they are the most reliable indicators of your hydration requirements.

Hydration significantly influences cognitive performance, enhancing focus and memory retention. This is crucial for tasks demanding high concentration, from important presentations to daily work routines. Research in the Human Brain Mapping Journal demonstrates that adequately hydrated individuals show more efficient brain function, particularly in areas related to planning and problem-solving. This efficiency not only boosts professional productivity but also enriches personal life, making the simple act of drinking water a powerful tool for improving mental agility and overall performance.

So, how can you ensure adequate hydration throughout the day? It's not just about drinking eight glasses of water. Innovations in how we consume water can make hydration an enjoyable and refreshing part of your daily routine. Infusing water with fruits, vegetables, or herbs is a fantastic way to enhance its flavor naturally, making it more appealing if you find plain water too bland. Try combinations like cucumber and mint or berries and lemon for a refreshing twist. These infusions not only make the water taste better but also add vitamins and antioxidants, boosting your nutrient intake. Another method is to set regular reminders on your phone or computer, prompting you to take hydration breaks. This can be especially useful if you tend to lose track of time during busy workdays.

Embracing these hydration strategies can significantly boost your physical stamina and mental acuity. Understanding the critical importance of water for both your body and mind, and finding creative methods to meet your hydration needs, turns the simple act of drinking water into a seamless and powerful tool for enhancing your overall health and well-being.

Planning Meals for Energy and Focus

When it comes to maintaining high energy levels and sharp focus throughout your bustling day, what you eat, when you eat, and how you balance your nutrients play pivotal roles. Let's break down the strategies and types of food that can transform your meal planning from a routine chore to a powerful tool for boosting your daily productivity and mental clarity.

Starting with the right foods is crucial. Certain items are known not just for their nutritional value but for their ability to enhance energy and concentration. For example, oats are a fantastic breakfast choice due to their high fiber content, which provides a steady release of energy into your bloodstream. This avoids the mid-morning crash that more sugary breakfast options can cause. Pairing oats with a protein source like Greek yogurt or a handful of nuts can further enhance their energy-stabilizing effect. Similarly, leafy greens such as spinach and kale are packed with iron, an essential mineral that helps in energy production and oxygen circulation in the blood. A lack of iron can lead to fatigue and reduced cognitive function. Including these greens in a lunchtime salad or smoothie can help keep your energy levels optimal.

Timing your meals can also significantly impact your energy and focus. The goal is to prevent the large spikes and dips in blood sugar levels that not only lead to energy crashes but also affect your concentration and productivity. Eating smaller, more frequent meals is a strategy that works well for many. For instance, instead of three large meals, breaking your food intake into five or six smaller meals can keep your metabolism active and maintain steady blood sugar levels. This could look like having a mid-morning snack of almonds and a banana between breakfast and lunch, followed by a mid-afternoon snack of hummus and carrots before dinner. This strategy can be particularly effective if your lifestyle includes irregular hours or high physical activity, as it provides continuous energy and helps in muscle recovery and repair.

Incorporating slow-release energy foods into your diet is another key strategy. Foods that are high in complex carbohydrates, such as whole grains, legumes, and starchy vegetables, provide a slower and more sustained release of energy.

This is due to their complex structures, which take longer to break down during digestion, providing a gradual supply of glucose into your bloodstream. For someone who has long days either at the office or managing home responsibilities, integrating these foods can prevent the lethargy that often hits mid-afternoon. A lunch that includes quinoa, chickpeas, and a variety of vegetables dressed with olive oil provides a balanced mix of complex carbohydrates, protein, and healthy fats, keeping you satiated and focused into the evening.

Let's put all this together into a sample meal plan that balances energy intake across the day, tailored to a typical busy lifestyle. Imagine starting your day with a breakfast of overnight oats prepared with almond milk, and chia seeds, and topped with fresh berries. This meal kicks off your day with a rich mix of fiber, protein, and antioxidants. Mid-morning, you could snack on a small handful of nuts to keep your energy up until lunch. For lunch, a quinoa salad with mixed greens, sliced avocado, and grilled chicken offers a perfect combo of complex carbs, healthy fats, and protein. Come mid-afternoon, when energy levels might typically start to wane, a green smoothie can give you a quick, nutrient-packed pick-me-up without the heaviness of more solid food. Finally, a dinner of grilled salmon with sweet potato and steamed broccoli rounds out the day with a meal high in omega-3 fatty acids, complex carbs, and essential nutrients, supporting both your brain function and overall health.

By understanding and implementing these principles of energy-boosting foods, optimal meal timing, and the incorporation of slow-release energy foods, your meal planning can effectively support both your energy levels and cognitive function, making every meal a step toward a more energetic and focused you.

Integrating Nutritional Strategies with Family Dining

Bringing balanced nutrition into the heart of family life not only enriches the dining table but also fosters lifelong healthy eating habits for everyone, from the smallest to the eldest. The challenge, of course, lies in preparing meals that cater to diverse tastes and nutritional needs without chaining you to the kitchen all day. Let's start with some family-friendly healthy recipes that are as nutritious as they are delectable, and designed to appeal to all age groups. For instance, a one-pan dish like baked salmon with a side of roasted carrots and potatoes can be a hit. It's rich in omega-3 fatty acids, beta-carotene, and essential minerals, covering a broad spectrum of nutritional needs while keeping the cooking and cleaning minimal.

Educating children about nutrition is another vital component. It's about making mealtime both fun and informative, turning it into an opportunity for kids to learn about what's on their plate. Why not let them be 'chef for a day'? With supervision, kids can help with simple tasks like rinsing veggies or mixing ingredients. During these activities, chat about the benefits of each ingredient, like how tomatoes are full of vitamin C, which helps keep their immune system strong. This not only helps children understand the value of good food but also makes them more likely to eat what they've helped prepare.

Dealing with different dietary preferences in a single household can be quite the tightrope walk. However, it's entirely possible to satisfy various palates and requirements without having to cook multiple distinct meals. Start by preparing versatile base dishes that can be customized according to individual preferences. For example, a vegetarian stir-fry can be served as is for those avoiding meat, or you can quickly sauté some chicken on the side for the carnivores in the family. This approach keeps everyone's taste buds happy and ensures that meal preparation remains straightforward and stress-free.

Encouraging healthy eating habits within the family setting goes beyond just serving nutritious meals. It involves creating a dining environment that promotes a positive attitude towards food. Regular family meals are a fantastic way to model healthy eating behaviors. When children see their parents enjoying a variety of foods, they are more likely to emulate those choices. Moreover, use mealtime as a chance to disconnect from screens and connect with each other. This not only improves digestion but also strengthens family bonds, making meals a nurturing experience for the body and soul.

In integrating these nutritional strategies into your family dining, you're doing more than just feeding the body; you're nurturing a foundation of wellness that can support your loved ones throughout their lives. By offering balanced meals, educating young ones about nutrition, accommodating various dietary needs, and fostering healthy eating habits, you turn the family table into a place of health, joy, and connection.

In wrapping up this exploration of family-focused nutrition, remember that the goal is to create a supportive eating environment that respects individual needs while promoting collective health. The strategies discussed here are designed not just to nourish but to inspire, bringing a sense of well-being that extends beyond the dinner table and into every aspect of life. As we close this chapter and move forward, the focus will shift to another crucial aspect of holistic health that often goes unnoticed—sleep. The next chapter will delve into how quality sleep is not just a pillar of good health but a foundation for vitality and well-being, exploring strategies to enhance sleep quality for you and your family.

"Proper nutrition fuels both the mind and body, creating a foundation for overall well-being and vitality."

Chapter 2 Wellness Plan: Nutrition for the Mind and Body

Activity: Daily Nutrition Reflection

Morning
- ★ What did you have for breakfast?
- ★ How did it make you feel (energized, sluggish, satisfied)?

Midday
- ★ What did you have for lunch?
- ★ Did you include any fruits or vegetables?

★ How did it impact your focus and energy in the afternoon?

Evening

★ What did you have for dinner?

★ Did you balance your proteins, fats, and carbohydrates?

★ How did it affect your overall well-being?

Reflection Questions:

★ *Which meal made you feel the best and why?*

★ *What changes can you make to improve your daily nutrition?*

Meditation: Mindful Eating (5 minutes)

★ *Sit in a quiet place with a small, healthy snack (like an apple slice or a few nuts).*

★ *Take a few deep breaths to relax.*

★ *Observe the texture, color, and smell of your snack.*

★ *Take a small bite, chew slowly, and notice the flavors and sensations.*

★ *Reflect on how mindful eating can enhance your appreciation and enjoyment of food.*

Suggested Music:

★ **Classical Piano:** *Chopin's Nocturnes, Op. 9*

★ **Nature Sounds:** *Forest or ocean waves*

Take a few minutes each day to jot down your reflections and notice any patterns in how your food choices impact your energy and focus. Use meditation to cultivate a habit of mindful eating.

Chapter 3

Physical Fitness in a Busy World

Picture this: it's early morning, you've just wrapped up a brisk workout, and you're feeling more alive and ready to tackle the day than ever before. Sounds ideal, doesn't it? Yet, for many of us juggling the demands of work, family, and personal commitments, regularly fitting in exercise can seem like a lofty goal. However, what if the key isn't finding more time but rather making the most of the time you do have with a flexible, tailored fitness routine that evolves with your lifestyle? That's exactly what we're diving into in this chapter—creating a fitness plan that not only fits into your busy schedule but also sparks joy and boosts your energy levels, making it a sustainable part of your daily life.

Designing a Flexible Fitness Routine

Assessing Personal Fitness Goals

Begin by assessing what you hope to achieve through your fitness routine. Goals in fitness are as varied as the individuals setting them. You might aim to build strength, enhance cardiovascular health, lose weight, or simply maintain your current fitness level. It's important to align these goals with your overall lifestyle and health status. Consider factors like your work schedule, family responsibilities, and any health conditions that might influence the type of activities best suited for you. For instance, a high-intensity workout might be perfect for a single professional looking to blow off steam after a busy day at the office, whereas a parent juggling work and kids might find more success with shorter, more frequent workouts that can be easily paused and resumed.

Creating a Modular Workout Plan

Once you have your goals in place, the next step is to create a workout plan that's as flexible as your week might be unpredictable. This is where the concept of a modular workout plan comes into play. Think of your weekly exercise routine as a collection of building blocks, each block representing a different activity that can fit into various time slots throughout your week. For instance, you might have a 30-minute block for a quick run, a 20-minute block for a yoga session, and even shorter 10-minute blocks for full-body stretches or quick high-intensity interval training (HIIT) sessions. The key is to develop a variety of these blocks that can be mixed and matched depending on how much time you have on any given day. This approach not only keeps your routine flexible but also prevents boredom and burnout, as you're not stuck doing the same workout every day.

Variety and Enjoyment

Speaking of variety, it's crucial for keeping your fitness journey enjoyable and effective. Incorporating different types of activities not only keeps things interesting but also ensures that you're working different muscle groups and giving others time to rest and recover. This could mean cycling between cardiovascular exercises, strength training, flexibility workouts, and balance exercises. Each type of exercise offers unique benefits and keeps your body guessing, which can help to prevent plateaus in your fitness progress. Moreover, consider what activities you actually enjoy. If you love being outdoors, make sure to include outdoor jogs or cycling in your routine. If you prefer group settings, a weekly dance class or a sports team meet-up might be the ticket to sustaining your fitness motivation.

Technology Aids

In today's digital age, technology offers a plethora of tools that can help you plan and track your workouts effectively. Fitness apps like MyFitnessPal or Strava not only help you monitor your physical activities but also provide insights into your progress, offer new workout ideas, and even connect you with a community of like-minded individuals for that extra dose of motivation. Wearable devices such as fitness trackers and smartwatches can be particularly useful, tracking everything from your step count and heart rate to your sleep patterns and recovery needs. These devices make it easier to stay on top of your fitness goals and adjust your routine as needed based on real-time data about your body's performance and needs.

By dedicating time to evaluate your fitness objectives, crafting a workout regimen that embraces flexibility, and leveraging technology for guidance and tracking, you pave the way for a fitness routine that seamlessly aligns with your dynamic lifestyle. This strategy guarantees a fulfilling and enjoyable path towards physical wellness, intricately woven into the fabric of your daily routine. It empowers you to enjoy the fruits of robust health and energy, ensuring your well-being thrives amidst the demands of life.

Home Workouts That Fit Your Life

Turning your home into a gym might sound like a daunting task, especially if you're short on space or don't have specialized equipment. But it's surprisingly feasible to create effective workout areas within the confines of your living space, using what you already own. Let's explore how you can transform your living area into a flexible gym that accommodates your fitness routine, no matter the size of your home.

For those working with limited space, the key is to utilize multi-functional furniture and areas that can easily be converted into workout zones. A yoga mat can turn any small space into a spot for yoga or pilates, and when you're done, it rolls up and tucks away. If you're looking to do more strength training, using sturdy furniture like a heavy chair or a low, stable table can substitute for gym equipment. For example, chairs can be excellent props for performing tricep dips or incline push-ups. Even a wall can be invaluable for exercises like wall sits or for stabilizing during a standing yoga pose. The idea is to look at your home not just as a place of rest but as a potential dynamic gym that you can maneuver around and adapt based on your workout needs.

Bodyweight exercises are a fantastic way to build strength and endurance without any equipment. Exercises like push-ups, sit-ups, planks, and squats are classics for a reason—they work. But beyond these basics, there are variations that can keep your routine engaging and challenging. For instance, switching from a regular squat to a single-leg squat can dramatically increase the intensity of the workout, targeting different muscle groups and improving balance. Introducing a routine of bodyweight exercises can be done in sequences or circuits, providing cardiovascular benefits alongside strength training, all from the comfort of your living room or bedroom.

In the digital age, you're never exercising in isolation, even from home. A wealth of online resources, including HIIT, dance, yoga, and strength training classes, are available at your fingertips through platforms like Peloton and apps such as Nike Training Club. These digital platforms not only provide a variety of workout options but also foster a community, offering connection and motivation to keep you consistent and engaged. Whether a beginner needing direction or an advanced user craving new routines, these online classes cater to all fitness levels.

By reimagining your living space, incorporating bodyweight routines, utilizing online resources, and involving the whole family, staying fit at home becomes not just an achievable goal but a sustainable and enjoyable part of your daily routine. These strategies ensure that your journey to fitness is as flexible and integrated into your lifestyle as it is beneficial to your health and happiness, proving that you don't need a gym membership to stay in shape and feel great.

High-Intensity Interval Training (HIIT) for Time-Savers

Imagine squeezing the most out of every workout minute, maximizing your fitness results without having to spend hours at the gym. That's the core premise of High-Intensity Interval Training or HIIT, a training technique that combines short bursts of intense exercise with periods of rest or lower-intensity exercise. The beauty of HIIT lies in its efficiency, making it an ideal workout for those who find it challenging to carve out extensive daily time for exercise. This method leverages the power of intensity to deliver significant cardiovascular and metabolic benefits in less time than traditional workout regimes.

The structure of a HIIT workout is simple yet incredibly effective. It alternates between periods of pushing your body to its max and allowing brief recovery times. For example, a typical session might involve 30 seconds of sprinting followed by 30 seconds of walking; this cycle is then repeated several times. Each burst of strenuous activity ramps up the heart rate, pushing the cardiovascular system to tap into energy reserves through anaerobic breathing. This not only improves heart health but also boosts metabolism, encouraging the body to burn more calories not just during the workout, but also for hours after.

To get you started, here's a sample HIIT routine that can be completed in just about 20-30 minutes and is adaptable to various fitness levels. Beginners might start with intervals of less intense activities like brisk walking alternated with moderate jogging. Those more advanced could opt for sprinting intervals interspersed with bodyweight exercises like squats or push-ups. Here's how you might structure it:

◆ Warm-up: 5 minutes of light jogging or a brisk walk to get your heart rate up.

◆ Cycle: 1 minute of sprinting followed by 1 minute of walking or light jogging, repeated 10 times.

◆ Cool down: 5 minutes of gradual slowing down of activity and stretching.

One of the most compelling benefits of HIIT is its ability to enhance cardiovascular health while effectively reducing body fat. The vigorous exertion required pushes the heart to pump faster, strengthening the cardiovascular system over time. Moreover, the intensity of the workout increases the metabolic rate, which means your body continues to burn calories at a higher rate even after you have finished exercising. This effect, known as the 'afterburn,' can be particularly beneficial for those looking to lose weight or improve their body composition.

Incorporating HIIT into your weekly routine can be seamlessly done, even with a tight schedule. Because these workouts are so efficient, you can fit them into various parts of your day. Morning person? Try a quick session first thing in the morning to kickstart your metabolism. More of a lunchtime exerciser? A 30-minute HIIT workout can be an excellent way to break up your day, leaving you energized for the afternoon. Even if your day is broken up with meetings or childcare responsibilities, HIIT's flexibility allows you to get a full workout in short, manageable segments, making it easier to maintain your fitness regimen without disrupting your daily responsibilities.

By embracing HIIT, you're not just saving time; you're also committing to a highly effective, scientifically backed method that enhances your health, accelerates fat loss, and boosts your endurance. Whether you're a busy professional, a parent managing a household, or someone simply looking to maximize their workout efficiency, HIIT offers a powerful solution to fit exceptional exercise into a compact time frame, ensuring you stay on track with your fitness goals regardless of your busy lifestyle.

The Role of Walking: Underrated Exercises

Walking, often overlooked in the rush for trendy high-intensity workouts or specialized fitness regimes, holds remarkable benefits for health that cater to all ages and fitness levels. Regular walking strengthens the heart, reduces the risk of cardiovascular disease, and helps manage weight by boosting the metabolism. Furthermore, it's an excellent mood enhancer; stepping out for a walk on a sunny day can significantly uplift your spirits thanks to the natural endorphins released during physical activity. The simplicity of walking, coupled with its profound impact on health, makes it an ideal, low-barrier entry point for anyone looking to improve their physical and mental well-being.

Incorporating more walking into your daily routine can be surprisingly straightforward and requires little adjustment to your existing schedule. If you commute to work, consider getting off a bus or train stop earlier and walking the rest of the way. Alternatively, if you drive, parking further away from your office can provide a good brisk walk that wakes you up before the workday starts and helps you decompress on your way home. Lunch breaks also offer a perfect opportunity; a quick 10-15 minute walk after eating not only aids digestion but also helps avoid the post-lunch energy dip. For those working from home, setting reminders to take brief walking breaks can be beneficial. These short bursts of activity not only break the monotony of prolonged sitting but also enhance circulation and mental alertness.

With today's digital tools, monitoring your walking achievements is effortless. Fitness trackers and smartphone apps track steps, distance, and calories, making it simple to set and achieve daily or weekly goals. These goals offer a clear sense of progress and accomplishment. Engaging in app-based challenges or with friends adds a fun, motivational aspect to your routine, encouraging you to remain dedicated and consistently push your boundaries.

To enhance your walking routine and keep it interesting, consider varying your routes and trying different walking techniques. Interval walking, which involves alternating between fast and moderate paces, can improve your cardiovascular health in a way that's similar to interval training. Adding weights, like a weighted vest or ankle weights, can increase the intensity of your walks, building strength and endurance. Choosing paths with varied elevations or terrains challenges different muscle groups, enhancing balance and flexibility. These simple changes can diversify your walking routine, amplifying its health benefits and making every step count.

Walking, often underrated, is a versatile physical activity accessible to all. It's an ideal choice for enhancing health gently, without the intensity of rigorous exercise regimes. Integrating walking into daily life, along with tools for tracking progress and diversifying routines, offers extensive health benefits. It keeps exercise interesting and manageable, regardless of your fitness level. Walking is the perfect low-impact step to enrich your wellness journey.

Combining Fitness with Family Time

Integrating fitness into family life not only strengthens the body but also the bonds between family members, creating shared experiences that are both healthy and joyful. Picture a sunny Saturday morning where instead of scrolling through phones, the entire family is out cycling through the park, laughing and racing each other, or perhaps an evening where everyone winds down with a friendly game of soccer in the backyard. These activities do more than just burn calories; they build memories and strengthen relationships. Activities like hiking, cycling, and playing sports are not only fantastic ways to get everyone moving but also opportunities for teaching teamwork, respect for nature, and the joy of living an active life.

The benefits of incorporating fitness activities that the whole family can participate in are immense. For children, these activities help instill a love of exercise from an early age, setting the foundation for healthy lifestyle habits. For adults, it's a way to model healthy behavior and stay active, which can be especially challenging given the demands of parenting and careers. Moreover, when families engage in physical activities together, they experience a unique type of bonding. This shared experience can enhance communication, foster mutual support, and provide a sense of accomplishment that strengthens familial ties. Additionally, regular physical activity has been shown to improve mental health and emotional well-being for all ages, reducing symptoms of anxiety and depression and elevating mood.

Scheduling regular physical activities for the family requires some creativity and flexibility, especially with varying schedules and interests. One effective strategy is to establish a routine that incorporates physical activity into the weekly schedule. This could be as simple as designating Sunday afternoons for family hiking trips or setting aside time every evening after dinner for a walk around the neighborhood. The key is consistency and making sure these activities are viewed as fun and enjoyable rather than another chore on the list. It can also be helpful to involve the whole family in the planning process, allowing each member to choose activities. This not only ensures that the activities align with everyone's interests but also increases the commitment level of all family members.

Leveraging family fitness time as a learning moment adds significant value. While hiking, for example, parents can introduce children to various plants and animals, seamlessly integrating a science lesson into the exercise. Sports activities can become practical lessons in fair play, teamwork, and resilience. Discussing the health advantages of these activities instills in children the importance of being active, fostering a lifelong positive outlook on health and fitness. These discussions not only enrich the family's wellness knowledge but also make the shared experience more enriching. Such moments are pivotal in building a resilient, health-conscious family unit, transforming fitness from an individual undertaking into a collective journey of joy and well-being.

Overcoming Common Physical Activity Barriers

When it comes to maintaining a regular exercise routine, it's not uncommon to hit a few roadblocks along the way. Whether it's the struggle to find time, waning motivation, or physical constraints, these barriers can often derail even the best-laid fitness plans. However, recognizing and understanding these obstacles is the first step toward overcoming them and achieving your fitness goals.

Identifying Personal Barriers

The first step in overcoming any obstacle is to identify it clearly. For many, time constraints are a major barrier, with days filled from morning to night with work, family duties, and social obligations leaving little room for exercise. Others might find that motivation ebbs and flows unpredictably, making it hard to stick to a routine. Physical limitations, whether due to an injury, chronic condition, or general fitness level, can also pose significant challenges. By pinpointing exactly what's holding you back, you can tailor your approach to tackle these specific issues head-on. For instance, if time is your biggest challenge, tracking how you spend your day might reveal hidden pockets of time that could be dedicated to physical activity.

Strategies to Overcome Barriers

Once you've identified your barriers, the next step is to develop strategies to navigate around them. Planning workouts ahead of time can be incredibly effective, especially for those who struggle with time management. At the start of each week, look at your schedule and block out times for physical activity, treating them as fixed appointments just like any other important commitment. For motivation issues, setting small, achievable milestones can help maintain a sense of progress and accomplishment. Celebrating these small victories can provide a continuous boost to your motivation levels. Additionally, finding a workout buddy or joining a fitness group can offer the necessary encouragement and accountability to keep you on track. The social aspect of exercising with others can transform your workout from a chore into an enjoyable social activity.

Adapting Exercises for Physical Limitations

For those dealing with physical limitations, adapting exercises to fit your abilities is key. Many exercises can be modified to accommodate different levels of mobility or strength. For example, if you have knee problems, you might switch from high-impact activities like running to lower-impact options such as swimming or cycling, which provide cardiovascular benefits without excessive strain on your joints. Resistance training can be adjusted by changing the weight, the number of repetitions, or even the speed of execution to better suit your capabilities. Consulting with a physical therapist or a certified fitness trainer who can provide personalized advice and modifications can ensure that you not only avoid injury but also make the most of your workout sessions.

Building a Support System

Finally, building a support system can play a crucial role in maintaining your motivation and commitment. This network can include friends, family, fitness professionals, or even online communities that share your fitness goals and challenges. Sharing your goals and progress with this group can make the journey less daunting and more supported. Whether it's having a friend to remind you of your workout appointments, family members who encourage you to stay on track, or a personal trainer who tailors your exercise program to your evolving needs, each component of your support system serves to keep you motivated and focused on your fitness goals.

By actively addressing each barrier with specific, tailored strategies, you can transform the way you approach physical activity. It becomes less about finding time or motivation and more about creating a lifestyle that naturally incorporates fitness into your daily routine. With each small step, whether it's a modified exercise to suit your physical condition or a quick workout squeezed into a busy day, you're building a foundation for lasting health and wellness that respects both your body's needs and your life's demands.

The Importance of Rest and Recovery

In the rhythm of push and pull that characterizes a well-rounded fitness regimen, the value of rest and recovery cannot be overstated. Often, the enthusiasm to achieve physical goals leads us to overlook these critical components, yet they are as vital as the workouts themselves. Rest days are essential in any fitness plan as they allow muscles to repair, rebuild, and strengthen. More importantly, they help prevent injuries that could otherwise set you back significantly. During high-intensity workouts, muscle fibers undergo stress and develop small tears. It's during the recovery period that these fibers heal and grow stronger, preparing your body to handle similar stress in the future more efficiently. This cycle of stress and recovery ultimately leads to physical improvements, making rest an indispensable part of training.

Recognizing the signs of overtraining is crucial in maintaining a healthy balance in your fitness journey. Symptoms like persistent muscle soreness, feeling drained instead of energized after a workout, insomnia, irritability, and a plateau or decline in performance can all indicate that your body needs more rest. These signals should not be ignored as they are your body's way of communicating that it cannot cope with the demands being placed on it. Listening to these signs and adjusting your training accordingly is essential to prevent burnout and injury. Remember, more is not always better; sometimes, the best thing you can do for your body is to allow it time to rest and recover.

Active recovery plays a pivotal role in any fitness routine by promoting recovery without overexertion. Techniques such as yoga, stretching, and light walking keep the body moving and blood circulating, which helps in reducing muscle stiffness and speeding up the healing process. Yoga, for instance, combines physical postures with breathwork and meditation, aiding in muscle and mental relaxation while improving flexibility and balance. Similarly, a gentle walk or a light cycle session can invigorate your muscles without the intensity of a full workout. These activities provide the benefits of keeping you physically active and engaged while still supporting the recovery process.

The deep connection between sleep and physical performance is essential. Quality sleep is crucial for recovery, as the body repairs muscles and releases growth hormones during deep sleep. To enhance sleep quality—and, consequently, recovery—try establishing a consistent bedtime, creating a quiet, dark sleeping environment, and avoiding caffeine before bed. Sleep-tracking apps can also help optimize your rest. Better sleep not only supports physical recovery but also boosts cognitive function and mood, enhancing your overall fitness journey.

Incorporating rest and recovery strategies, acknowledging signs of overtraining, engaging in active recovery, and prioritizing good sleep hygiene is crucial for a successful fitness regimen. They enable sustainable training, enhancing physical strength and overall well-being. As this chapter concludes, remember that rest days and recovery periods are as vital as the workouts themselves. Embracing this balance safeguards your health and propels you towards achieving your fitness goals with vitality and resilience.

As we transition from understanding the foundational elements of physical fitness, the focus will shift toward mental, emotional, and spiritual wellness in the upcoming chapters. These facets are intricately linked with our physical state and exploring them will provide a more holistic view of what it means to live a truly healthy life.

> *"Even in a busy world, physical fitness is essential; it nourishes the body, sharpens the mind, and enriches the spirit."*

Chapter 3 Wellness Plan: Physical Fitness in a Busy World

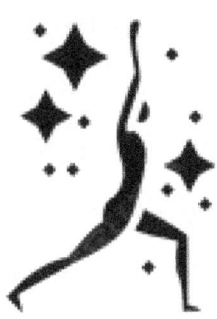

Activity: Reflective Exercise

Take a moment to reflect on your current approach to physical fitness in the context of your busy lifestyle. Consider the barriers you face, the strategies you've used to overcome them, and any areas where you feel there's room for improvement. Then, jot down your thoughts in a journal or notebook. Here are some prompts to guide your reflection:

1. **Identify Your Barriers:** *What are the main obstacles preventing you from maintaining a consistent fitness routine? Are they related to time, motivation, physical limitations, or something else entirely?*

2. **Strategies for Overcoming Barriers:** *Reflect on the strategies you've implemented to overcome these bar-*

riers. Which ones have been most effective for you? Are there any new approaches you'd like to try?

3. **Reflect on Progress:** *Take stock of your progress so far. What achievements are you proud of? What challenges have you encountered, and how have you worked through them?*

4. **Future Goals:** *Based on your reflections, what are your goals for improving your physical fitness moving forward? How do you plan to integrate these goals into your busy lifestyle?*

Music Suggestions:

★ **Energetic Playlist:** *Curate a playlist of high-energy songs that get you pumped up and ready to tackle your workouts. Include upbeat tracks from your favorite artists or explore new genres to find tunes that inspire movement and motivation.*

★ **Instrumental Relaxation:** *Wind down after a workout or during moments of reflection with soothing instrumental music. Choose calming melodies or ambient sounds that promote relaxation and rejuvenation, helping you recharge for the next phase of your journey.*

Once you've completed your reflection and chosen your music selections, take a moment to acknowledge the effort you've put into prioritizing your health and well-being. Remember, progress is a journey, and every step forward, no matter how small, is a victory worth celebrating.

Chapter 4

Mental, Emotional, and Spiritual Health Nourishment

Imagine your mind as a serene landscape, where thoughts flow like a gentle river, emotions bloom like vibrant flowers, and your spirit soars like the wind above. Sounds idyllic, doesn't it? Yet, for many of us, this mental landscape often feels more like a stormy sea than a tranquil garden. The challenges of balancing demanding careers, family responsibilities, and personal aspirations can stir up stress, anxiety, and a host of emotional upheavals. However, nurturing your mental, emotional, and spiritual health is as crucial as maintaining your physical well-being—perhaps even more so, as it forms the core from which our overall health radiates. This chapter is dedicated to equipping you with practical, accessible strategies to cultivate a resilient, peaceful mind and a nourished spirit, transforming your mental landscape into the serene haven you envision.

Practical Mindfulness Exercises for Anxiety

Breathing Techniques

One of the most immediate ways to temper anxiety is through mindful breathing, which can shift your body's response to stress from a state of alarm to one of calm. Techniques like the 4-7-8 breathing method, developed by Dr. Andrew Weil, are particularly effective. Here's how you do it: breathe in quietly through your nose for 4 seconds, hold your breath for 7 seconds, and exhale forcefully through your mouth, pursing your lips and making a "whoosh" sound, for 8 seconds. This method serves as a natural tranquilizer for the nervous system, slowing your heart rate and calming your mind. Another powerful technique is box breathing, used by Navy SEALs to stay calm and focused. It involves inhaling to a count of four, holding your breath for four seconds, exhaling for four seconds, and holding again for four seconds, forming a box pattern. Practicing these breathing exercises daily, or whenever anxiety begins to creep in, can help you regain control of your emotions, grounding you in the present moment.

Mindful Observation

When anxiety levels rise, turning your focus outward can help diminish their grip. Mindful observation involves selecting any object in your immediate environment and noting every detail about it. It could be a tree you pass by every day, a book on your coffee table, or simply a cup of coffee. Observe the colors, textures, shapes, and even the way light interacts with the object. This practice helps anchor your mind in the now, diverting it from anxious thoughts about the past or future, and fostering a serene attentiveness that can refresh and reset your emotional state.

Guided Visualizations

Guided visualizations are a form of mental escape that can provide powerful relief from anxiety. By mentally transporting yourself to a peaceful setting—say, a quiet beach at sunset or a cool, dark forest—you engage your mind in creating calming sensations that can overpower anxious thoughts. You can find guided visualization scripts online or through meditation apps like Calm or Headspace, which guide you through scenic narratives designed to engage your senses and transport you to tranquility.

Mindfulness Meditation

Integrating simple mindfulness meditation into your daily routine can significantly enhance your ability to manage anxiety. This practice involves sitting quietly and paying attention to your thoughts, breathing, or sensations in your body without judgment. Every time your mind wanders, gently bring it back to your focus point—be it your breath, a word, or a phrase. The key is consistency; even five to ten minutes a day can make a profound difference. Over time, mindfulness meditation increases your awareness of the present moment, allowing you to catch anxious thoughts before they spiral and address them with a calm, centered mind.

Through these practical exercises—breathing techniques, mindful observation, guided visualizations, and mindfulness meditation—you can cultivate a toolkit that empowers you to navigate the ebbs and flows of mental and emotional tides with grace and resilience. The beauty of these practices lies in their simplicity and accessibility, making it possible for anyone, regardless of their hectic schedule or life demands, to integrate them into daily life, paving the way toward a more peaceful, mindful existence. As we continue to explore the various dimensions of mental, emotional, and spiritual wellness, remember that each step you take on this path enriches not just your own life but also the lives of those around you, creating ripples of positivity and health that extend far beyond the immediate.

Cognitive Behavioral Techniques Without the Jargon

Identifying Cognitive Distortions

Navigating the maze of your thoughts can sometimes feel like a daunting task, especially when negative thinking patterns begin to cloud your judgment. Cognitive distortions, simply put, are ways that our mind convinces us of something that isn't really true. These inaccurate thoughts usually reinforce negative thinking or emotions, telling us things that sound rational and accurate, but really only serve to keep us feeling bad about ourselves. For instance, 'all-or-nothing' thinking leads you to view everything at extremes with no middle ground, while 'catastrophizing' involves expecting the worst-case scenario to happen. Recognizing these patterns is the first step in managing them. When you catch yourself thinking "I didn't finish this project perfectly, I'm a failure," that's all-or-nothing thinking. Start by simply noticing these thoughts and labeling them. This awareness creates a mental space between you and your reactions, providing a moment to choose how you respond.

Challenging Negative Thoughts

Once you identify these distortions, the next step is to challenge and reframe them into more balanced thoughts.

This is where you question the validity of your negative thoughts and replace them with more positive and accurate ones. It's like being a detective examining the evidence for and against your established way of thinking. For example, if you're thinking, "I will never be good at this," ask yourself, "What evidence is there to support this?" Most likely, you'll find that there are past instances where you have succeeded or made significant improvements. By methodically disputing these negative thoughts, you gradually diminish their power over your emotions and begin to see a more realistic picture of yourself and your abilities.

Behavioral Activation

Behavioral activation is a tool for overcoming depression and anxiety by encouraging you to engage in activities that you find meaningful and enjoyable. It operates on the principle that doing pleasant activities, particularly those that align with your values, can improve your mood and reduce feelings of anxiety. Start by making a list of small activities that bring you joy or a sense of satisfaction. This could be anything from reading a book, taking a walk in nature, or playing a musical instrument. The key here is consistency and gradually increasing the frequency of these activities. Over time, as you engage more in these fulfilling activities, you'll likely find a shift in your mood and outlook, breaking the cycle of negativity that feeds depression and anxiety.

Journaling for Cognitive Change

Journaling is a powerful tool for cognitive restructuring, offering a way to track your thoughts and patterns over time. By keeping a daily log of your feelings and the thoughts that accompany them, you begin to uncover patterns and triggers in your thinking. Use your journal to apply the cognitive techniques you've learned: write down distressing thoughts, identify the distortions, and challenge them. Over time, this practice can lead to significant shifts in how you perceive and react to the world around you. It's a personal reflection space where you can openly explore your emotions and the cognitive processes influencing them, fostering a deeper understanding and mastery over your mental health.

By employing cognitive behavioral techniques, you gain practical tools to transform your mental landscape. Identifying and correcting distorted thinking, engaging in activities that lift your mood, and journaling for reflection fosters a positive and fulfilling mental state. These strategies not only improve your mental and emotional health but also encourage proactive steps towards a more balanced lifestyle. As we delve deeper into mental and emotional wellness strategies, remember that each action you take is a step towards a clearer, more serene mind.

Building Resilience Against Daily Stressors

Developing a Resilience Mindset

In your daily life, stressors can range from small annoyances to large challenges. Developing a resilience mindset is like constructing a dam to control stress, preventing it from overwhelming you. It's not about dodging stress but learning to navigate through it. This mindset is built on acceptance, growth, and positivity. Acceptance means recognizing stress as an inevitable part of life, thereby reducing the tension that comes from resisting it. Growth involves viewing challenges as opportunities to learn and enhance your abilities, encouraging a proactive stance towards stress. Positivity, the third pillar, shapes your stress response, helping you find the good in situations, maintain high spirits, and adopt a problem-solving attitude.

Stress Inoculation Training

Stress Inoculation Training (SIT) is a technique designed to bolster your ability to manage stress by gradually exposing you to it in a safe, controlled way—similar to how vaccines build immunity. This method unfolds in three stages: understanding stress and your reactions to it, learning and practicing stress management skills like relaxation and positive thinking, and then applying these skills in increasingly challenging situations. For example, to conquer a fear of public speaking, you might begin by talking to yourself in the mirror, then move on to presenting in front of a small group of friends, and finally, speak at larger, more formal events. This step-by-step exposure helps diminish the anxiety and fear tied to stressors, thereby strengthening your resilience.

Routine Building

Creating a daily routine is a powerful strategy to mitigate stress by introducing structure and predictability into your life. By identifying the core elements of your day—such as meal times, work, exercise, and family interactions—and organizing your schedule around these, you decrease the mental burden of decision-making and the stress of unforeseen events. This structure provides a sense of control and efficiency, acting as a shield against stress. It's essential, however, to weave relaxation and leisure into this framework to ensure ongoing self-care and stress management. Additionally, a well-considered routine can stabilize your biological clock, leading to better sleep and higher energy levels. Remember, the essence of a beneficial routine lies in its flexibility; it should accommodate spontaneous needs and adjustments, preventing the rigidity from becoming a stressor itself.

Support Networks

The strength of a support network is invaluable in reducing stress. Comprising family, friends, colleagues, or support groups, it offers emotional solace and practical assistance when needed. Opening up to trusted individuals not only eases your emotional burden but also brings fresh perspectives and solutions. It counters the isolation stress often brings. Professionally, sharing tasks and solutions or just having someone who listens can be a significant relief. Building these connections demands mutual effort and trust, involving active participation in community events, clubs, or online groups, thereby broadening your support circle and fortifying your resilience.

These resilience-building strategies are crucial in your journey to holistic wellness. By cultivating a resilient mindset, engaging in Stress Inoculation Training, establishing a balanced daily routine, and fostering a robust support network, you empower yourself to navigate life's challenges more smoothly. These steps not only improve your current stress management but also arm you for future hurdles, promoting sustained health and fulfillment. As we delve deeper into mental, emotional, and spiritual wellness, remember that these strategies are interconnected, each enhancing the other towards a harmonious and enriched life.

Managing Social Anxiety Through Small Steps

Navigating social landscapes can often stir a whirlpool of anxiety for many, turning simple interactions into daunting challenges. If you find yourself feeling tense before a social event or rehearsing conversations in your mind long after they've ended, you're not alone. Tackling social anxiety doesn't have to be an overwhelming leap; small, manageable steps can significantly ease the journey, making social interactions less intimidating and more enjoyable. Let's explore some gentle yet effective strategies designed to help you build confidence and reduce anxiety in social settings.

<u>Gradual Exposure</u>

The concept of gradual exposure is a cornerstone in managing social anxiety. It involves slowly and systematically confronting social situations that you find anxiety-inducing, rather than avoiding them. Start with less challenging interactions, such as saying hello to a neighbor or asking a store clerk a question, and gradually work your way up to more anxiety-provoking scenarios like attending a large gathering or giving a presentation. Each exposure opportunity allows you to experience and handle anxiety in a controlled manner, which over time, can help diminish the intensity of your reactions to these situations. It's like dipping your toes in the water before diving in; each step builds your confidence and reduces the fear associated with social interactions.

Social Skills Training

Improving your social skills can also play a significant role in alleviating social anxiety. Basic training in this area might include learning effective conversation starters or practicing active listening skills. For starters, try commenting on a shared situation or environment, like remarking on the weather or a piece of artwork at an event. This not only breaks the ice but also provides a mutual topic for discussion. Active listening, where you focus fully on the speaker, nodding and responding appropriately, can help you engage more deeply in conversations, making interactions more meaningful and less stressful. These skills don't just ease anxiety; they enhance your ability to connect with others, enriching your social experiences.

Role-playing Exercises

Role-playing is another invaluable tool in your arsenal against social anxiety. It allows you to rehearse social scenarios in a safe, non-threatening environment, typically with a therapist or a trusted friend. By simulating a social interaction and practicing your responses, you can gain confidence and reduce anxiety about real-life encounters. For instance, role-playing a job interview with a friend can help you practice answers to common questions, reducing anxiety when you face the actual situation. Over time, these rehearsals can help desensitize you to the stressors of social interactions, making them feel more manageable and less intimidating.

Self-Compassion Exercises

Cultivating self-compassion is crucial, especially when dealing with anxiety in socially challenging situations. Practice exercises that foster kindness and understanding toward yourself, particularly when you feel you've fallen short in social interactions. One effective method is to write yourself a letter from the perspective of a compassionate friend. In this letter, address yourself with kindness, acknowledge your feelings, and offer encouragement. This exercise helps shift your perspective, reducing self-criticism and fostering a gentler, more forgiving view of your social performances.

Professional Help

Lastly, if social anxiety significantly impacts your ability to function in professional or personal settings, seeking professional help can be a vital step. Therapists specializing in anxiety disorders can provide guidance and support through proven techniques like Cognitive Behavioral Therapy (CBT) or Acceptance and Commitment Therapy (ACT). These therapies offer structured approaches to understanding and managing your anxiety, providing tools and strategies that are tailored to your specific needs. Additionally, support groups for social anxiety can also be beneficial, offering a platform to share experiences and learn from others facing similar challenges.

By approaching social anxiety with these small, structured steps—gradual exposure, social skills enhancement, role-playing, self-compassion practices, and professional guidance—you can navigate social landscapes with increasing ease and confidence. Each step not only builds your social skills but also reinforces your ability to manage anxiety, transforming daunting social interactions into opportunities for connection and growth. As you continue to apply these techniques, remember that progress in managing social anxiety is a gradual journey, marked by small victories and continuous learning. Each effort you make is a building block in constructing a more confident, socially engaged version of yourself, paving the way for richer, more fulfilling interactions.

Enhancing Sleep Quality for Emotional Well-being

Understanding how closely sleep is intertwined with your emotional and mental health can be a game-changer in managing stress and enhancing your overall life satisfaction. It's a two-way street: just as emotional stress can lead to sleep disturbances, poor sleep can exacerbate stress, creating a cycle that can be hard to break. Deep, restorative sleep, on the other hand, acts much like a reset button for the brain, allowing you to process emotional experiences and regulate mood more effectively. During the REM (Rapid Eye Movement) stage of sleep, your brain actively processes and consolidates emotions and memories from the day. If sleep is cut short or frequently interrupted, you miss out on this critical processing time, which can lead to more pronounced emotional reactions and a decreased ability to cope with stress. Moreover, a lack of adequate sleep is linked to a higher risk of conditions such as depression and anxiety. Prioritizing good sleep is not just about physical rest—it's about giving your brain the chance to heal, reset, and strengthen.

Sleep Hygiene Practices

Establishing effective sleep hygiene is key to improving your sleep quality. Consider sleep hygiene as the foundation of good sleep practices. A consistent sleep schedule is vital—aim to go to bed and wake up at the same time daily, reinforcing your natural sleep-wake cycle. Equally important is a pre-sleep routine to calm your mind, such as reading, taking a warm bath, or engaging in gentle yoga or deep breathing exercises. Creating a sleep-friendly environment is also crucial. Your bedroom should be a haven for rest: ensure it's comfortable, quiet, dark, and kept at a cooler temperature. Quality bedding and the use of blackout curtains or an eye mask can further enhance your sleep setting.

Tools for Better Sleep

In our modern, tech-savvy era, leveraging tools and technologies can greatly enhance sleep quality. Wearable devices like Fitbit and apps like Sleep Cycle offer insights into your sleep habits by monitoring movements and heart rate to track sleep stages, including REM sleep. This information allows for personalized adjustments to improve sleep patterns. Additionally, white noise machines can create a tranquil environment by emitting soothing sounds such as rain or ocean waves, masking external disturbances and promoting uninterrupted sleep.

Addressing Common Sleep Disturbances

Many people grapple with sleep disturbances stemming from stress-induced insomnia and disruptive environmental conditions. Techniques aimed at calming the mind, such as progressive muscle relaxation—which involves tensing and then relaxing muscle groups—and mindfulness meditation, can significantly mitigate the mental unrest that hampers sleep. Furthermore, addressing environmental disruptors is essential. Ensuring your sleep haven is dim, quiet, and cool, with the ideal temperature around 65 degrees Fahrenheit, can profoundly enhance sleep quality. Incorporating blackout curtains and white noise machines also helps in creating an optimal sleep environment conducive to restful nights.

By embracing these practices and tools—maintaining consistent sleep patterns, creating a conducive sleep environment, using technology to enhance sleep quality, and addressing common disturbances—you can significantly improve your sleep quality. This, in turn, supports your emotional and mental health, making it easier to manage daily stresses and maintain a balanced mood. As we continue to explore more aspects of mental, emotional, and spiritual well-being, remember that sleep is not just a period of inactivity; it's an active and vital process of renewal and healing, crucial for a vibrant, joyful life.

Tech Tools That Aid Mental Wellness

In an era where technology permeates almost every aspect of our lives, it's no surprise that it also offers tools to help manage our mental wellness. These innovations come in various forms, from apps that ease the symptoms of anxiety to wearable devices that help monitor our physiological states. Embracing these tools can provide a significant boost to managing everyday mental health challenges, making psychological well-being more accessible and manageable, especially for those balancing busy schedules.

Mental health apps, such as Headspace and Calm, are revolutionizing the way we manage stress and anxiety through guided meditations and sessions tailored to various needs and schedules. These platforms, including Moodpath, offer mood tracking and daily check-ins to monitor your emotional well-being, helping to identify patterns or triggers. Incorporating these apps into your routine—starting with a few minutes of meditation each morning, for instance—can significantly improve your emotional stability and set a positive tone for your day.

Wearable technology, such as Fitbit and Apple Watch, significantly aids mental wellness by monitoring heart rate variability (HRV), a crucial stress and emotional arousal indicator. These devices track your physiological state, enhancing your awareness of stress levels and suggesting when to pause for calming activities. For instance, an elevated heart rate signal could prompt you to take a moment for deep breathing or a brief walk. This immediate feedback is essential for effective stress management, allowing timely interventions to prevent overwhelming situations.

The rise of online therapy platforms like BetterHelp and Talkspace has dramatically increased access to professional counseling. These services offer text, voice, or video calls, making mental health support more convenient for those with hectic schedules or limited access to local services. With a wide selection of therapists, these platforms cater to a variety of needs, enhancing the accessibility and flexibility of receiving guidance for minor to moderate mental health issues. Virtual Reality (VR) technology presents a fresh approach to managing phobias and anxiety disorders. It simulates fear-triggering scenarios in a safe, controlled environment, allowing individuals to face their fears with a therapist's support. For example, VR can mimic flight experiences for those with a fear of flying, enabling them to practice coping strategies safely. The immersive quality of VR offers a unique and effective form of exposure therapy, serving as a practical alternative to facing fears in real life. With its growing accessibility, VR holds significant promise for personalized mental health interventions, marking an innovative step forward in therapeutic practices.

By integrating these technological tools into your mental health care strategy—whether through apps, wearable devices, online therapy, or VR—you can enhance your ability to manage stress, anxiety, and other mental health challenges more effectively. These tools offer practical, accessible solutions that fit into your lifestyle, empowering you to take control of your mental wellness in a way that feels tailored and responsive to your needs. As we continue to navigate the complexities of modern life, these technologies serve as valuable allies in our quest for mental and emotional balance, making the journey a little smoother and the load a little lighter.

Art and Music Therapy: Creative Outlets for Stress Relief

Engaging in art and music can be profoundly therapeutic, serving not only as outlets for creativity but also as effective tools for stress relief and emotional management. The act of creating art or enjoying music stimulates the release of endorphins, the body's natural feel-good chemicals, promoting relaxation and joy while reducing stress and anxiety. This process can help elevate your mood, boost your self-esteem, and provide a sense of accomplishment. Whether you're painting, drawing, playing an instrument, or just listening to your favorite tunes, the arts offer a unique pathway to tranquility and emotional balance that can be especially beneficial in today's fast-paced, often stressful environment.

Getting Started with Art Therapy

For those new to art as a form of therapy, the beginning can be as simple as grabbing a piece of paper and some colored pencils. Art therapy isn't about creating masterpieces; it's about expressing yourself and finding emotional release through the creative process. Start with simple activities like doodling or coloring in an adult coloring book. These activities don't require you to be artistically skilled but can provide a focus for your mind, drawing it away from stressors and allowing a meditative calmness to take over. If you feel more adventurous, try your hand at clay modeling or watercolor painting, which can be incredibly soothing and rewarding. Local community centers or art schools often offer classes that can provide structured guidance and introduce you to various materials and techniques. The key is to focus on the process rather than the outcome, letting your creativity flow freely without judgment.

Integrating Music into Daily Routine

Music's power to influence our emotions and mood is nearly universal, making it a fantastic tool for managing stress and enhancing well-being. To incorporate music into your daily life, consider creating playlists that resonate with different moods or activities. A playlist with calming, soothing tunes is perfect for unwinding after a stressful day, while an upbeat, energetic playlist can be motivating during a workout or when tackling household chores. If you play an instrument, setting aside time each day to play can be not only an enjoyable skill to cultivate but also a powerful stress reliever. Even if you don't play an instrument, simply sitting back and actively listening to music, allowing yourself to fully experience and engage with the sounds, can be a therapeutic practice. It can help center your thoughts and calm your mind, much like meditation.

Case Studies and Success Stories

The transformative power of art and music therapy is supported by numerous success stories. For example, a young professional overcame burnout through painting, reconnecting with her passion for life and work. Similarly, a retired individual battling depression found solace and community through guitar lessons, which alleviated his loneliness. These examples underscore the dual benefits of art and music: they serve as effective forms of personal therapy and means of building connections, thereby boosting emotional well-being. Art and music therapy are not only accessible and enjoyable but also powerful ways to improve mental health and manage stress. Engaging in these creative practices can uplift your mood, foster personal growth, and enhance life satisfaction. As we conclude this chapter, we emphasize the importance of incorporating these creative outlets into our routine as part of a comprehensive approach to nurturing our mental, emotional, and spiritual health. The insights gained here pave the way for exploring more holistic wellness strategies in subsequent chapters, aiming for a balanced and fulfilling life.

> *"Nourishing your mental, emotional, and spiritual health is the cornerstone of holistic wellness, fostering inner peace and balanced living."*

Chapter 4 Wellness Plan: Emotional and Mental Wellness

Activity Reflective Exercise:

Mindfulness Reflection:

★ **Reflection:** Think about a recent moment when you felt emotionally or mentally balanced. What were you doing? How did it make you feel?

★ **Example:** "I felt very calm and content while taking a walk in the park last weekend. The fresh air and nature around me brought a sense of peace."

Embracing Positivity:

★ **Reflection:** Identify three positive affirmations that resonate with you and explain why they are meaningful.

★ **Example:** "I am resilient. This affirmation reminds me of my ability to overcome challenges and keep moving forward."

Wellness Rituals:

★ **Reflection:** Describe a daily or weekly ritual that helps maintain your emotional and mental wellness. How does it contribute to your overall well-being?

★ **Example:** "Every morning, I spend 10 minutes journaling my thoughts and intentions for the day. It helps clear my mind and sets a positive tone."

Emotional Check-In:

★ **Reflection:** Conduct a quick emotional check-in. Rate your current emotional state on a scale from 1 to 10 and describe why you chose that number. What can you do to improve or maintain this state?

★ **Example:** "Today, I feel like a 7. I'm generally happy, but a bit stressed about work deadlines. Taking short breaks and practicing deep breathing could help reduce the stress."

Music Suggestions:

Energetic Playlist:

Create a playlist of high-energy songs that boost your mood and motivation. Include tracks that inspire you to move and feel positive.

★ "Happy" by Pharrell Williams
★ "Uptown Funk" by Mark Ronson ft. Bruno Mars
★ "Can't Stop the Feeling!" by Justin Timberlake

Instrumental Relaxation:

Wind down with soothing instrumental music that promotes relaxation and calm. Choose melodies that help you relax after a busy day.

★ "Weightless" by Marconi Union
★ "Clair de Lune" by Claude Debussy
★ "Ambient 1: Music for Airports" by Brian Eno

Acknowledge Your Effort:

Take a moment to acknowledge the effort you've put into prioritizing your emotional and mental well-being. Reflect on one thing you are proud of achieving in your wellness journey. Celebrate this progress, no matter how small it might seem. Remember, every step forward is a victory worth celebrating.

Chapter 5

Spiritual Growth and Personal Faith

Imagine starting your day not with the blare of an alarm and a mad dash to get ready, but with a moment of peace, a sacred ritual that grounds you and sets a serene tone for the challenges ahead. In a world that often values productivity over tranquility, dedicating time to nurture your spiritual self can seem like a luxury. However, integrating spiritual practices into your daily routine can profoundly impact your emotional resilience, mental clarity, and overall sense of well-being. This chapter invites you to explore simple yet profound daily practices that can enhance your spiritual growth and enrich your life's tapestry, no matter how hectic your schedule might seem.

Daily Practices for Spiritual Growth

Establishing a Morning Routine

Setting the tone for your day can significantly influence your mindset and productivity. Incorporating spiritual practices such as prayer, meditation, or reading spiritual texts each morning can provide a foundation of peace and purpose. Imagine this routine as your personal sanctuary time—undisturbed, quiet moments where you connect with something greater than the day's to-do list. This might look like spending a few minutes in meditation, reflecting on a passage from a spiritual book, or simply sitting in silence, savoring the stillness before the day unfolds. These practices aren't just about spiritual enlightenment; they're about setting a deliberate, mindful tone for your day, giving you a reservoir of calm to draw from when stress and challenges arise.

Gratitude Journaling

In the rush of daily responsibilities, it's easy to focus on what's going wrong or what's missing. Shifting this focus to gratitude can dramatically alter your perception, enhancing both your spiritual and emotional well-being. Maintaining a gratitude journal is a simple yet powerful practice to cultivate this mindset. Each day, take a few moments to write down things you are grateful for. These don't have to be grand revelations; often, it's the small comforts and joys—like a delicious cup of coffee, a child's laughter, or a comforting chat with a friend—that fill our lives with meaning. This practice trains your mind to recognize and appreciate these moments, enriching your life experience and elevating your spirit.

<u>Mindful Breathing</u>

Breathing, often an automatic action, becomes a potent spiritual tool when done with intention. Practicing deep diaphragmatic breathing—inhaling deeply through the nose to expand the abdomen, pausing, then exhaling slowly through the mouth or nose—can center your spirit, calm the mind, and anchor you in the present. This simple exercise reduces stress and restores clarity and composure, seamlessly integrating mindfulness into moments of stress or decision-making.

<u>Incorporating Spirituality in Work and Relationships</u>

Spirituality transcends the boundaries of solitary reflection, infusing every facet of our daily lives with depth and meaning. Introducing brief meditative breaks throughout the workday can rejuvenate your mental clarity and enhance concentration, transforming routine tasks into opportunities for mindfulness. Similarly, practicing attentive listening and presence during conversations with colleagues and loved ones not only fosters deeper connections but also promotes a mutual exchange of respect and understanding. By integrating spirituality into both mundane and meaningful activities, you create a life imbued with intention and awareness, thereby enriching your interactions in the professional sphere and personal relationships alike.

Meditation and Its Varieties: Finding What Fits

Meditation, often envisioned as a monk in serene silence on a mountain peak, is actually a versatile and widely accessible practice that can be adapted to fit into the bustling lives of anyone—from a busy CEO to a stay-at-home parent. The beauty of meditation lies in its diversity; numerous types cater to different preferences and objectives. Take mindfulness meditation, for example, which immerses you in the now, fostering an environment of mindfulness and acceptance. It's ideal for anyone eager to dial down stress levels and boost their focus. Conversely, transcendental meditation relies on mantra repetition to usher in profound relaxation and tranquility, making it a perfect fit for individuals in search of a more guided form of meditation.

Guided visualization is another form of meditation where you are led through a series of visualizations to promote relaxation and mental clarity. This type can be especially appealing if you find it challenging to focus or if you are a visual learner. Lastly, loving-kindness meditation focuses on developing feelings of compassion and love towards oneself and others. It's a powerful practice for fostering positivity and reducing negative emotions like anger and resentment. Each type of meditation offers unique benefits and can be a tool for personal growth and wellness, depending on what you feel you need most in your life.

Incorporating meditation into your life need not be time-consuming. A brief session of five to ten minutes each day can bring significant benefits. Optimal times for meditation include during your morning routine, on a lunch break, or just before sleep. For those commuting, guided audio meditations can turn travel time into a moment of restoration. The key to experiencing the full benefits of meditation lies in regular practice, making it a natural and impactful part of your daily health regimen.

Adopting a variety of meditation practices into your routine transcends basic relaxation and concentration techniques. It unlocks access to a profound toolkit for enhancing every facet of your existence. Whether your quest involves seeking serenity, mental clarity, a profound spiritual bond, or emotional resilience, meditation offers a tailored pathway to achieve your unique aspirations. Integrating meditation into your daily schedule transforms it from a mere activity to a cornerstone of your wellness journey. Embark on this exploration with an open heart and consistent effort, letting your personal affinities lead the way. This method cultivates a sense of equilibrium, peace, and a profound connection with the here and now.

The Role of Nature in Spiritual Wellness

Stepping outside, feeling the breeze on your face, hearing the rustle of leaves underfoot, and seeing the sunlight filter through the trees can transform an ordinary day into an extraordinary moment of connection with the natural world. The benefits of spending time in nature are not just physical; they extend deeply into our spiritual and psychological well-being. Nature has a unique ability to heal, soothe, and restore us, often just by our simply being present within it. Engaging with the natural environment can significantly lift our spirits, enhance mindfulness, and reduce stress. This connection is rooted in our very makeup; humans evolved in natural settings, and despite modern life's pull toward urban environments, our affinity for nature remains profound.

For those looking to deepen their spiritual connection through nature, several activities can foster this bond. Hiking, for instance, offers more than just physical exercise; it provides an opportunity to experience the quiet majesty of nature, which can be a profound spiritual experience. Each step taken on a forest trail can be a step deeper into mindfulness, where the mind is focused, the heart rate slows, and the hustle of daily life fades away. Gardening goes beyond simple beauty, serving as a meaningful path to self-care and growth. Planting each seed represents a commitment to what lies ahead, and the diligent nurturing of plants reflects the fostering of one's growth and patience.

Walking barefoot on grass, a practice known as "earthing" or "grounding," imbues the body with a natural tranquility, alleviating stress and enhancing well-being. This simple act of connecting physically with the earth is a powerful reminder of our bond to the natural world, offering an immediate sense of peace and groundedness. Such experiences underscore the profound impact nature has on our spiritual and psychological health, serving as a sanctuary away from the modern urban lifestyle.

Nature itself can be a profound teacher, offering lessons on resilience, change, and interconnectedness. Observing the natural cycles of growth, decay, and rebirth can provide deep insights into the nature of our own lives. For example, watching a river persistently flow towards the sea can teach us about perseverance and the importance of following our course. Witnessing a tree stand tall through the seasons, enduring storms, and basking in sunlight, can remind us of the strength and flexibility required to face life's various challenges. These lessons, when contemplated, can enhance our understanding of life and our place within it, enriching our spiritual journey.

Creating sacred spaces in natural settings can further enhance this connection. Whether it's a corner of your backyard, a spot under a favorite tree in a local park, or a quiet place by a nearby lake, these spaces can serve as sanctuaries for meditation, reflection, and connection. You might consider placing objects that hold personal significance in these spaces or creating altars with natural elements like stones, plants, and water. These acts of personalization make the space uniquely yours, a physical manifestation of your spiritual connections to nature. Spending time in your sacred space, surrounded by the elements of the natural world, can be incredibly restorative and uplifting.

In embracing the natural world as part of your spiritual practice, you open yourself to a wellspring of peace, clarity, and connectedness. These experiences in nature not only provide a respite from the stress of daily life but also deepen your spiritual existence, offering a broader perspective and a renewed sense of wonder and gratitude for the world around you. As you continue to explore and integrate these practices into your life, you may find that your time spent in nature becomes essential to your spiritual wellness, a vital part of your path to inner peace and fulfillment.

Creating a Personal Ritual for Spiritual Health

Rituals are the threads that weave the fabric of our spiritual lives, offering both a structure to navigate the chaos of daily living and a profound means to celebrate life's milestones, both big and small. In a world that often prizes spontaneity and flexibility, the deliberate and thoughtful nature of rituals can provide a comforting sense of stability and continuity. These sacred acts serve as anchors, grounding us in our beliefs and values amidst the ebbs and flows of life. Whether it's a simple morning routine of lighting a candle and setting intentions for the day, or a complex ceremony marking personal milestones like birthdays or anniversaries, rituals remind us of who we are and what matters most to us. They create a rhythm to our lives that nurtures our spiritual health and bolsters our resilience against the unpredictability of the world.

Creating personal rituals that resonate with your beliefs and needs doesn't require adherence to rigid rules or elaborate preparations; rather, it's about crafting meaningful practices that reflect your individuality and support your spiritual journey. Start by identifying moments in your life that you feel deserve recognition or need special attention—perhaps a time of transition, like starting a new job or moving to a new home, or moments that call for healing, such as recovering from illness or loss. Once you've pinpointed these moments, think about actions that hold significant spiritual or emotional weight for you. This could involve writing down affirmations, planting a tree, or even preparing a special meal. The key is to imbue these actions with intention and mindfulness, transforming them into powerful acts of ritual that celebrate or soothe the soul.

Choosing symbols or artifacts that carry personal significance can enhance the power of your rituals. These objects act as visual and tactile anchors for your intentions, imbuing your practice with depth and focus. For instance, a particular stone picked up from a place you feel connected to can serve as a symbol of strength or stability. Similarly, photographs of loved ones might represent love and connection, serving as focal points in rituals that honor relationships. The sounds used during your rituals—whether chants, prayers, music, or simple silence—can also significantly affect the atmosphere, helping to transport you to a state of deeper contemplation or celebration.

Sharing your personal rituals with a community can be profoundly enriching. It not only strengthens individual spiritual practices but also fosters a sense of shared experience and mutual support. Imagine a ritual where friends or family gather to share stories of gratitude, each person lighting a candle to symbolize their thanks. Such practices create bonds of understanding and empathy, reinforcing community ties and providing a collective strength that supports each member's spiritual growth. Engaging with others in ritual practice not only deepens relationships but also expands your own spiritual perspectives, allowing you to experience the diverse expressions of faith and spirituality within your community.

Faith Across Cultures: Universal Wellness Lessons

In the rich tapestry of global cultures, diverse spiritual traditions converge on common grounds—teachings of compassion, mindfulness, and forgiveness. These principles, deeply embedded in the doctrines of major world religions, form a universal blueprint for wellness that transcends geographical and cultural boundaries. For instance, Buddhism teaches the practice of mindfulness and loving-kindness to cultivate peace within oneself and towards others. Christianity emphasizes forgiveness and love, with the principle of treating others as one would like to be treated oneself. Similarly, Islam promotes compassion and mindfulness through daily prayers and the practice of Zakat, or charity, which fosters a sense of empathy and responsibility towards the less fortunate.

Delving into these foundational teachings enriches our comprehension and underscores our collective desire for connection and purpose. It unveils how, despite diverse rituals and expressions, the core of our moral and spiritual wellness is strikingly alike. Such insights are enlightening for those on spiritual paths or deepening their grasp of humanity and spirituality. By embracing these universal truths, we access a treasury of knowledge that fortifies well-being, applying age-old wisdom to contemporary life, thus enhancing our spiritual journey.

Appreciating the diversity of spiritual paths enriches your own spiritual journey. It opens up a myriad of perspectives and practices that can invigorate your faith or spiritual practice with new insights and methodologies. For example, engaging with the Islamic practice of daily reflection, or Muhasaba might inspire you to incorporate regular self-assessment into your spiritual routine. Alternatively, the Jewish tradition of Sabbath observance, a day dedicated entirely to rest and spiritual enrichment, could encourage you to define clear boundaries for work and relaxation, enhancing your work-life balance and spiritual growth.

These interfaith explorations foster not only personal growth but also a deeper social understanding, promoting tolerance and respect in increasingly multicultural societies. By learning about and respecting diverse religious practices, you contribute to a more empathetic world where spiritual diversity is celebrated as a strength rather than feared as a divide. This approach not only broadens your spiritual horizons but also models a pathway for others in your community, promoting a culture of mutual respect and curiosity.

Moreover, integrating elements from various faiths into your personal spiritual practice should be approached with sensitivity and respect. It's essential to engage with these elements authentically and considerately, ensuring that your adoption of foreign practices is both respectful and meaningful. Start by learning deeply about the context and significance of the practices you wish to adopt. Engage with communities and leaders within those faith traditions, seeking guidance and understanding to ensure that your practices honor their origins and intentions. This respectful integration enriches your spiritual life, not only with diverse practices but also with a profound respect and appreciation for the beliefs of others, fostering a personal spirituality that is both inclusive and expansive.

As you weave these interfaith insights and practices into your life, you create a mosaic of spiritual wellness that is both deeply personal and expansively global. This approach does not dilute your beliefs but rather deepens them, allowing you to stand firmly in your faith while reaching out with openness and respect to the myriad of ways humanity seeks and finds meaning. In doing so, you contribute to a world where spiritual diversity is seen as an invaluable resource for wisdom, peace, and deep, universal wellness.

The Benefits of Spiritual Retreats in Everyday Settings

Spiritual retreats serve as serene sanctuaries for deep reflection and rejuvenation, delivering profound impacts that surpass their peaceful surroundings. They grant a pause from the relentless pace of daily existence, inviting a journey into greater self-awareness and spiritual discovery. Engaging in these retreats can profoundly deepen your comprehension of your own identity and life's purpose, providing designated moments to step back from habitual activities and forge a closer connection with your core being. These immersive experiences often catalyze valuable revelations that propel personal development, emotional restoration, and a refreshed life orientation.

Exploring the different types of retreats can open up a world of tailored experiences that cater to your specific spiritual needs. Silent retreats, for example, emphasize the power of silence as a tool for deep meditation and self-reflection, allowing participants to turn their attention inward without the distraction of conversation. In contrast, meditation retreats focus on deepening participants' practice and understanding of meditation, often incorporating various techniques to aid spiritual growth and mental clarity. Yoga retreats offer a blend of physical and meditative practices that aim to harmonize body and mind, enhancing both physical health and spiritual well-being. Choosing the right retreat involves assessing your current spiritual needs and goals. For instance, if you're looking to find peace in times of stress, a silent retreat might provide the tranquil environment necessary for profound mental and emotional rest.

Creating mini-retreats at home is a practical way to incorporate the benefits of spiritual retreats into your daily life without the need to travel or take extended time off. Designating specific days or weekends for focused spiritual practices can create a retreat-like atmosphere in the comfort of your own home. This might involve turning off electronic devices, engaging in extended meditation sessions, or spending time in reflective reading and journaling. By setting aside dedicated time for these activities, you create sacred spaces and periods that allow for deep self-exploration and rejuvenation, mirroring the restorative experience of a traditional retreat.

Incorporating the serenity and revelations from retreat experiences into your routine is essential for sustained spiritual growth and fortitude. This may include adopting daily rituals that mirror the insights gained, such as engaging in morning meditations or setting aside time for introspection.

Chapter Conclusion

In this chapter, we explored the enriching world of spiritual growth through daily practices, diverse meditation techniques, and the transformative power of nature and personal rituals. Each section offered practical strategies to deepen your spiritual connections and enhance your overall well-being, emphasizing the importance of integrating these practices into everyday life. As we transition to the next chapter, we will build on these foundations, exploring holistic approaches to maintaining physical health, mental clarity, and emotional resilience, ensuring a balanced and fulfilling lifestyle.

> *"True holistic wellness arises when spiritual growth intertwines with unwavering personal faith, creating a balanced and fulfilling life."*

Chapter 5 Wellness Plan: Spiritual Growth and Personal Faith

Activity Reflective Exercise:
Establishing a Morning Routine:

★ **Reflection:** Think about your current morning routine. How can you incorporate a simple spiritual practice to start your day with peace and purpose?

★ **Example:** "I will start my mornings with 10 minutes of meditation, focusing on my breath and setting positive intentions for the day."

Gratitude Journaling:

★ **Reflection:** Each day, write down three things you are grateful for. Consider how this practice impacts your spiritual and emotional well-being.

★ **Example:** "Today, I am grateful for the sunny weather, a kind gesture from a colleague, and a delicious meal."

Mindful Breathing:

★ **Reflection:** Practice mindful breathing for a few minutes each day. Reflect on how this practice helps center your spirit and calm your mind.

★ **Example:** "I noticed that mindful breathing helps me feel more present and reduces my anxiety, especially before important meetings."

Connecting with Nature:

★ **Reflection:** Spend time in nature and observe its beauty and tranquility. Reflect on how nature influences your spiritual growth and overall sense of well-being.

★ **Example:** "A walk in the park today made me feel connected to something larger than myself. The fresh air and sounds of nature brought me a sense of peace."

Creating Personal Rituals:

★ **Reflection:** Think about a personal ritual you can create that resonates with your spiritual beliefs and needs. It could be as simple as lighting a candle and setting an intention for the day.

★ **Example:** "I created a ritual of lighting a candle each evening and spending a few minutes in silent reflection. It helps me unwind and feel grounded."

Exploring Meditation Varieties:

★ **Reflection:** Try different forms of meditation, such as mindfulness, guided visualization, or loving-kindness meditation. Reflect on which type resonates most with you and why.

★ **Example:** "Guided visualization helps me relax and focus. I enjoy the creative aspect of imagining peaceful scenes."

Incorporating Spirituality in Daily Life:

★ **Reflection:** Think about how you can integrate spirituality into your work and relationships. Reflect on the impact this has on your interactions and overall well-being.

★ **Example:** "I started taking brief meditative breaks at work and noticed an increase in my concentration and a decrease in stress. Being present during conversations with loved ones has deepened my relationships."

Learning from Different Faiths:

★ **Reflection:** Explore spiritual teachings from different cultures and religions. Reflect on the universal lessons and how they can enhance your spiritual journey.

★ **Example:** "Learning about the concept of mindfulness from Buddhism has taught me to be more present and compassionate in my daily life."

Personalizing Your Spiritual Path:

★ **Reflection:** Reflect on the unique aspects of your spiritual journey. Consider how you can honor and celebrate these aspects through personalized practices and rituals.

★ **Example:** "I personalized my meditation space with objects that hold special meaning to me, making it a sanctuary for spiritual reflection."

Acknowledging Your Effort:

After completing your reflections and implementing new spiritual practices, take a moment to acknowledge your dedication to your spiritual growth. Celebrate the small steps you've taken and the progress you've made. Remember, spiritual growth is a continuous journey, and every effort counts towards a more fulfilling and balanced life.

Music Suggestions:
1. **Uplifting Playlist:**
    ★ "Higher Love" by Kygo & Whitney Houston
    ★ "Rise Up" by Andra Day
    ★ "Here Comes the Sun" by The Beatles
2. **Relaxing Instrumentals:**
    ★ "River Flows in You" by Yiruma
    ★ "Gymnopédie No. 1" by Erik Satie
    ★ "Morning Mood" by Edvard Grieg

End of Chapter Reflection:

Reflect on the various practices you've explored in this chapter. How have they contributed to your spiritual growth and personal faith? Consider how you will continue to integrate these practices into your daily routine and the impact they have had on your overall well-being. As you move forward, continue to explore and refine your spiritual practices, allowing them to evolve and grow with you.

By engaging in these reflective exercises and incorporating the suggested practices, you can deepen your spiritual growth and enhance your personal faith, leading to a more balanced and fulfilling life.

Chapter 6

Sustainable Living and Wellness

Imagine if every choice you made in your daily routine could contribute not just to your personal health, but also to a healthier planet. From the soap you use to wash your hands to the clothes you pick out of your closet, every decision has the power to impact both your well-being and the environment. In this chapter, we dive into the heart of sustainable living and wellness, exploring how making eco-friendly choices can lead to a life that's not only healthier for you but also kinder to the world around you. It's about transforming our everyday habits into actions that nurture our health and cherish the planet—an approach that aligns perfectly with the holistic wellness principles we cherish.

Eco-Friendly Choices That Enhance Personal Health

In today's market, shelves are stocked with products claiming myriad benefits, yet many of these benefits don't extend to the environment. Switching to biodegradable and natural personal care products, such as soaps, shampoos, and toothpaste, is a simple yet effective way to reduce your exposure to potentially harmful chemicals while also minimizing your ecological footprint. These products are crafted to break down more easily in the environment, preventing pollutants from accumulating in our ecosystems. Moreover, they are often made without harsh chemicals, reducing the risk of skin irritations, allergies, and other health issues that can arise from synthetic ingredients. By choosing these products, you're not just cleansing your body; you're contributing to a cleaner, healthier environment.

The clothes we wear and the goods we consume also play a significant role in sustainable wellness. Opting for clothing made from organic cotton or recycled polyester not only reduces environmental damage (like pesticide use and waste accumulation) but also supports industries striving to reduce their carbon footprint. Wearing a shirt made from organic cotton, you're supporting farming practices that maintain soil health and reduce toxic pesticide usage. Similarly, choosing consumer goods made from recycled or sustainable materials helps decrease the demand for raw materials, which often involve environmentally intensive extraction processes. These choices ensure that your personal wellness journey contributes positively to the health of the planet, aligning your lifestyle with your values of care and responsibility.

Transportation is another area where you can make significant eco-friendly changes. Opting for greener methods such as biking, walking, or using public transit not only reduces your reliance on fossil fuels but also benefits your physical health. Regular physical activity, such as biking to work, can improve cardiovascular health, enhance mental well-being, and decrease stress levels. Moreover, using public transit can help reduce traffic congestion and the pollution that comes with it, leading to cleaner air and a healthier community. These transportation choices are integral to a sustainable lifestyle, promoting both environmental health and personal well-being.

Lastly, reducing energy consumption in your home through energy-efficient appliances, LED lighting, and smart thermostats not only cuts down on your utility bills but also your carbon footprint. Energy-efficient appliances use less electricity, which means less fossil fuel is burned in power plants, leading to fewer air pollutants that can cause respiratory problems and other health issues. Smart therapeutics allow you to control your home's heating and cooling systems more efficiently, avoiding unnecessary energy use and promoting a healthier indoor environment. By making these adjustments, you contribute to a larger movement of energy conservation, which is crucial for our planet's health and our own.

Embracing these eco-friendly practices represents a powerful step towards living a life that values sustainability and wellness. It's about making choices that respect and renew our resources—choices that ensure we not only thrive but so does the world around us. As we continue to explore more ways to integrate sustainable practices into our daily lives, remember that each small change we make is part of a much larger process of transformation—one that promises a healthier, more sustainable future for all.

Reducing Your Carbon Footprint with Smarter Food Choices

Eating is an everyday activity that inevitably impacts the environment, but it also holds fantastic potential for positive change. By making mindful choices about what you eat and how you manage food, you can significantly reduce your carbon footprint while improving your health. Let's explore how adopting practices like local and seasonal eating, embracing a plant-based diet, reducing food waste, and supporting sustainable farming can transform your meals into a powerful tool for environmental conservation and personal wellness.

Local and seasonal eating is not just a trendy concept; it's one of the most effective ways to enhance the quality of your diet while minimizing environmental impact. Foods grown locally require far less transportation, which significantly reduces carbon emissions associated with long-distance food transport. Additionally, seasonal produce tends to be fresher and more nutrient-rich, as it is harvested at its peak and doesn't require long periods in storage, where nutrients can degrade. This means that the strawberries you buy from your local farmer's market in June are likely to be tastier and healthier than those shipped from halfway across the world in December. By choosing local and seasonal foods, you also support the local economy and small farmers who are more likely to use sustainable practices that maintain soil health and biodiversity.

Transitioning to a plant-based diet is another powerful way to lower your carbon footprint. Livestock production is one of the largest contributors to environmental degradation, including deforestation, water scarcity, and greenhouse gas emissions. By reducing your consumption of animal products, you can help decrease the demand for these resource-intensive foods. A plant-based diet, which emphasizes vegetables, fruits, grains, and nuts, is not only environmentally sustainable but also beneficial for your health.

Studies have shown that it can reduce the risk of chronic diseases such as heart disease, hypertension, diabetes, and certain types of cancer. Moreover, plant-based diets often encourage a more creative approach to cooking and eating, inspiring you to explore a wider variety of foods and culinary techniques.

Food waste is a massive global issue, with significant environmental, economic, and social impacts. In the United States alone, it is estimated that about 30-40% of the food supply is wasted. This not only wastes the resources used for growing, transporting, and selling food but also contributes to methane emissions from landfills, a potent greenhouse gas. You can combat food waste by planning your meals ahead, buying only what you need, and storing food properly to extend its freshness. Learning how to use leftovers creatively is another skill that can reduce waste while adding variety to your meals. For instance, yesterday's roasted chicken can be today's chicken salad, and wilting vegetables can be transformed into a nutritious soup or stock.

Supporting farms and businesses that adhere to sustainable practices is crucial in promoting an environmentally responsible food system. Organic farming, permaculture, and other sustainable agriculture methods not only help reduce environmental impact but also produce healthier, more nutritious food. These practices avoid or significantly reduce the use of synthetic pesticides and fertilizers, which can contaminate water, soil, and even the food itself. By choosing products from farms that prioritize sustainability, you help create demand for these practices, encouraging more farmers to consider environmentally friendly options. Many communities now have farmer's markets, community-supported agriculture (CSA) programs, and local health food stores that offer direct access to sustainably produced goods. By making these choices, you not only ensure healthier food for yourself and your family but also contribute to a larger movement towards a more sustainable and equitable food system.

Each of these strategies offers a pathway to reducing your environmental impact while enhancing your health and supporting your community. Whether it's through choosing local produce, adopting a plant-based diet, minimizing food waste, or supporting sustainable farming practices, the choices you make at the dining table can have a profound impact on the planet. As you continue to explore and implement these practices, you'll find that eating sustainably can also be a delicious, rewarding, and deeply fulfilling experience.

Sustainable Fitness: Environmentally Conscious Exercise

Embracing the great outdoors for your fitness regimen not only revitalizes your body but also deeply reconnects you with nature, enhancing both your physical well-being and mental clarity. Imagine starting your day with a hike through a lush forest trail, the sounds of nature replacing the hum of gym machines, or perhaps kayaking on a serene lake, where the rhythmic splash of your paddle sets a meditative pace. Outdoor activities like hiking, cycling, and kayaking don't rely on electric power, which diminishes your carbon footprint and immerses you in natural settings that promote significant health benefits. These activities increase your exposure to vitamin D, enhance your mood through natural scenery, and improve your physical fitness by engaging different muscle groups in a dynamic environment. The psychological benefits are just as impactful, with natural settings shown to reduce stress, enhance mood, and improve overall mental health.

Switching to eco-friendly fitness gear can further align your exercise routine with sustainable practices. Consider yoga mats made from natural rubber or pilates equipment crafted from recycled materials. These choices not only reduce your ecological impact but also ensure that your health pursuits contribute positively to the environment. Similarly, opting for workout clothing made from organic cotton or recycled fabrics can significantly reduce the demand for new fibers, which often involve resource-intensive production processes. These materials offer the same functionality and comfort as their non-eco-friendly counterparts, ensuring that your transition to sustainable fitness gear is seamless and beneficial.

The community aspect of sports can also play a pivotal role in promoting both environmental sustainability and social well-being. Participating in community sports leagues often makes use of local fields and facilities, which helps reduce the need for long commutes to distant venues, cutting down on carbon emissions. These community-based activities foster a sense of belonging and teamwork, enhancing your social connections while engaging in physical exercise. The shared experience of playing sports can lead to stronger community bonds and a collective commitment to maintaining local recreational areas, which further supports environmental conservation efforts.

Lastly, if you're looking to simplify your fitness routine while minimizing your environmental impact, consider minimalist workouts that require little to no equipment. Exercises like push-ups, sit-ups, squats, and jogging are not only highly effective but also accessible to everyone, regardless of their location or economic status. These activities can be performed anywhere, from the smallest apartment to a local park, making it easier to fit exercise into your busy schedule without contributing to consumer culture through the purchase of equipment. This approach not only helps in maintaining physical fitness but also ensures that your workout regimen is sustainable, affordable, and inclusive.

By integrating these environmentally conscious practices into your fitness routine—embracing outdoor activities, choosing eco-friendly gear, participating in community sports, and adopting minimalist workouts—you create a fitness lifestyle that not only benefits your health but also contributes positively to the well-being of our planet. Each step you take in this direction supports a sustainable future while empowering you to live a healthier, more connected life. As you continue to explore and implement these practices, you'll find that sustainable fitness is not only about personal health but also about nurturing a deep respect and care for the environment we all share.

Household Toxins and Natural Alternatives

When you think about maintaining a healthy home, what often comes to mind is a space that's clean, well-organized, and inviting. But beneath the surface of shiny floors and polished countertops, there could be unseen threats lurking in the form of household toxins. Common substances like

BPA, phthalates, and formaldehyde are found in a myriad of household products, from plastic containers to furniture and air fresheners. These chemicals are not just bad for the planet; they can pose significant risks to your health, including hormonal disruptions and an increased risk of cancer. Awareness and proactive management of these substances can transform your home into a truly safe sanctuary.

Switching to natural cleaning products is a straightforward and effective way to reduce your exposure to harmful chemicals. Many everyday pantry items can be powerful cleaning agents; for instance, white vinegar and baking soda can handle everything from window cleaning to unclogging drains and polishing silver. For a simple all-purpose cleaner, mix equal parts of water and vinegar in a spray bottle and use it to wipe down surfaces — it's effective, safe, and economical. Adding a few drops of essential oils like lemon or lavender can provide a pleasant scent along with additional antibacterial properties. These natural alternatives not only keep your home clean but also ensure that you are not inhaling harmful chemical residues that can affect your health.

Maintaining good indoor air quality is crucial for a healthy home environment, especially considering how much time most people spend indoors. Regular use of salt lamps and beeswax candles can help in reducing airborne contaminants. Salt lamps attract and neutralize positively charged contaminants, improving air quality, while beeswax candles burn cleanly and emit negative ions that can bind with toxins and help remove them from the air. Additionally, incorporating air-purifying plants such as spider plants, snake plants, and peace lilies can bring a touch of nature indoors while filtering out pollutants and releasing oxygen.

Dealing with pests without resorting to harsh chemicals can be a challenge, but natural methods like diatomaceous earth, neem oil, and peppermint oil offer effective, non-toxic alternatives. Diatomaceous earth is a powder made from fossilized algae that is deadly to insects but harmless to humans and pets; it can be sprinkled in areas where bugs are a problem. Neem oil, derived from the seeds of the neem tree, works as a natural pesticide that disrupts the life cycle of pests without harming beneficial insects like bees and butterflies. Peppermint oil, aside from its pleasant scent, is a potent repellent for many types of insects, including spiders and ants. A few drops in water can be used to make a spray that, when applied to entry points, can keep your home pest-free naturally.

By identifying and mitigating common household toxins through natural cleaning products, improving indoor air quality, and using natural pest control methods, you can significantly enhance both your health and your environment. Each small change you make contributes to a healthier home and a healthier planet, aligning your lifestyle more closely with holistic wellness principles. As you continue to explore more ways to integrate natural alternatives into your daily routine, remember that each choice you make builds toward a safer, cleaner living space that nurtures both the body and the Earth.

The Wellness Benefits of Minimalism

The allure of a minimalist lifestyle is often portrayed in images of pristine living spaces bathed in white and sparse furnishings that promise a calm, uncluttered existence. But beyond aesthetics, adopting a minimalist approach can profoundly impact your mental health and overall well-being. Consider the experience of coming home to a cluttered space, where every surface is covered with unsorted mail, items from past shopping trips, and half-done projects. This visual chaos can trigger stress and anxiety, making it hard to find peace or focus. Now, imagine entering a space that contains only what you need and love—where there's room to breathe and space to relax. This environment can significantly decrease stress and anxiety levels, enhancing your ability to focus and process information more effectively.

The concept of conscious consumption, a cornerstone of minimalism, advocates for buying less but choosing well. It's about prioritizing quality over quantity, which naturally leads to less waste and a more sustainable lifestyle. This practice not only helps in reducing the clutter that can overwhelm your home and mind but also aligns your purchasing habits with your values, leading to a deeper sense of satisfaction and purpose. When you choose to buy a well-made product that lasts longer, you're not just making a purchase; you're making a statement about the kind of world you want to live in—one that values sustainability over disposability. This mindful approach to consumption can significantly reduce the environmental impact of your lifestyle, supporting a healthier planet as well as a more focused and value-driven personal life.

Creating minimalist living spaces is about more than discarding unwanted items; it's about designing environments that promote peace and functionality. Start by identifying the essentials, the items that serve a purpose or bring you joy, and let go of duplicates and those that no longer serve you. This doesn't mean your space has to be bare; rather, it should be curated thoughtfully to support your daily activities and personal aesthetics. For example, a bedroom might only have a bed, a wardrobe, and a couple of meaningful decorations that promote a restful ambiance. Such spaces are easier to maintain and clean, which reduces the time and stress associated with household chores, leaving more time for activities that enhance your well-being.

Digital minimalism is another facet of this lifestyle that can lead to significant improvements in mental and emotional health. In an age where digital clutter is as overwhelming as physical clutter, learning to streamline your digital engagement can free up time and reduce stress. Start by unsubscribing from emails that no longer serve you and limiting your exposure to social media, which can be a major source of anxiety and distraction. Instead, allocate time to digital activities that add value, such as educational podcasts or meaningful conversations with friends and family online. This approach helps reclaim your time and mental space from the demands of a constantly connected world, allowing for deeper engagement with the real world and a more balanced, fulfilling life.

Embracing minimalism in these various forms creates a lifestyle that is not only sustainable but also conducive to a deeper sense of peace and contentedness. It's about making more room for the things that truly matter—whether that's relationships, hobbies, or personal growth—and shedding the excess that distracts from these priorities. As you continue to explore and implement minimalist practices, you'll likely discover that this less-is-more philosophy isn't just about giving things up. It's about creating space for growth, peace, and fulfillment in ways that resonate with your personal values and lifestyle, enhancing both your well-being and the world around you.

Community Gardening and Local Food Sources

Embracing the concept of community gardening and supporting local food sources is not just about cultivating plants; it's about nurturing a community and fostering a connection to the earth that feeds us. Imagine stepping into a lush community garden, where every plot and plant tells a story of collaboration and care. Here, local residents, each with their own unique backgrounds and experiences, come together to sow seeds not only of vegetables and flowers but of friendship and mutual support. The benefits of participating in such a community initiative extend far beyond the harvest of fresh produce. They also include significant boosts to physical activity, as gardening is a wonderfully gentle yet effective form of exercise. Additionally, the mental health benefits are profound—gardening is known to reduce stress and promote feelings of well-being.

Starting a community garden might seem like a daunting task, but it can be broken down into manageable steps. First, securing a piece of land is crucial. This space could be a vacant lot, a rooftop, or even a series of large containers in a shared space. Once a location is secured, engaging community members is the next step. This involves reaching out to local residents, schools, and organizations to garner support and participation. Choosing what to plant can be a community decision as well, one that might depend on the local climate, the soil quality, and the preferences of the community gardeners. It's also essential to consider the maintenance and sustainability of the garden, which includes regular watering, weeding, and harvesting schedules that volunteers can sign up for. By breaking down the process and involving the community at every step, the garden becomes a collective endeavor where everyone's input and effort are valued.

Local food co-ops offer another avenue for supporting local farmers and accessing fresh, seasonal produce. In a food co-op, members buy shares of a farm's harvest in advance, providing farmers with the upfront funds needed to cover initial production costs. In return, members receive a regular share of the harvest throughout the farming season. This model not only ensures that farmers have a guaranteed market for their produce but also allows consumers to become intimately connected with the source of their food, often receiving items that are fresher and more varied than what's available in supermarkets. Moreover, many co-ops provide opportunities for members to visit the farms, meet the farmers, and even participate in farming activities, offering deeper insights into the food production process and fostering a greater appreciation for the labor and love that goes into growing food.

Community gardens and local food sources also serve as exceptional educational tools. They provide hands-on learning opportunities for people of all ages, teaching valuable skills in gardening, nutrition, and environmental stewardship. For children, participating in a community garden can be an enlightening experience, one that teaches them where food comes from and the importance of taking care of the environment. Adults, too, can learn a great deal about sustainable gardening techniques, seasonal food patterns, and the nutritional benefits of fresh produce. Furthermore, community gardens can host workshops and events focused on topics such as composting, plant identification, and cooking with garden-fresh ingredients, enhancing the educational benefits for all involved.

As this chapter on community gardens and local food sources concludes, reflect on how integrating these practices into your life might not only change the way you eat but also how you connect with others and engage with your environment. These initiatives offer a pathway to a more sustainable lifestyle, one that promotes health, supports local economies, and strengthens community ties.

As we move forward, the principles and practices explored here can serve as a foundation for a broader discussion on sustainable living, one that encompasses not only our food choices but also our daily habits and consumer behaviors.

"Holistic wellness is the harmony we cultivate within ourselves and with the world around us, and sustainable living is the pathway to achieving this balance."

Chapter 6 Wellness Plan: Sustainable Living and Wellness

Activity: Practical Sustainability

Take practical steps towards integrating sustainable living and wellness into your daily routine. Reflect on each activity, document your experiences, and explore how music can enhance your journey.

Eco-Friendly Product Audit:

◈ List your current personal care and household cleaning products.

◈ Research eco-friendly alternatives.

◈ Purchase and try one eco-friendly product.

☆ **Reflection:**

☆ How does the eco-friendly product compare to your usual one?

☆ *What differences did you notice in effectiveness or sensory experience?*

Sustainable Wardrobe Update:
◈ Identify three clothing items to replace with sustainable alternatives.
◈ Research brands offering sustainable materials.
◈ Purchase one sustainable clothing item.
☆ ***Reflection:***
☆ *How do you feel wearing the sustainable item?*
☆ *What did you learn about sustainable fashion?*

Greener Transportation Challenge:
◈ Use a green transportation method (walking, biking, public transit) for one day.
◈ Plan your route and schedule.
☆ ***Reflection:***
☆ *How did green transportation affect your physical health and mood?*
☆ *What challenges did you encounter and overcome?*

Energy Efficiency Check:
◈ Audit your home's energy usage (lights, appliances, heating/cooling systems).
◈ Identify three ways to reduce energy consumption (e.g., switching to LED bulbs).

- ◈ Implement one change.
- ☆ **Reflection:**
- ☆ What changes did you make and how easy were they to implement?
- ☆ Did you notice any immediate differences in your home environment?

Plant-Based Meal Prep:

- ◈ Plan and prepare three plant-based meals using local and seasonal ingredients.
- ☆ **Reflection:**
- ☆ How did the plant-based meals make you feel?
- ☆ Did you enjoy the process of cooking and eating these meals?

Minimalist Home Detox:

- ◈ Choose one area to declutter.
- ◈ Sort items into categories: keep, donate, recycle, discard.
- ◈ Organize the space.
- ☆ **Reflection:**
- ☆ How did decluttering affect your mental and emotional state?
- ☆ Did the process reveal any insights about your consumption habits?

Join or Start a Community Garden:
- ◈ Research community gardens or start one with a group.
- ◈ Spend one hour this week gardening.

☆ **Reflection:**
- ☆ What benefits did you experience from gardening (physical, mental, social)?
- ☆ How did it enhance your connection to the community?

Music Suggestions:

◈ **Energetic Playlist:**
- ☆ Curate a playlist of upbeat, motivational songs to energize you during eco-friendly product research or sustainable wardrobe updates. Include tracks that inspire action and positivity.

◈ **Calming Tunes for Reflection:**
- ☆ Create a playlist of soothing instrumental music or ambient sounds to play during your minimalist home detox or plant-based meal prep. Use calming melodies to promote relaxation and mindfulness.

Acknowledge Your Effort:

Take a moment to acknowledge the effort you've put into these activities. Reflect on the positive changes you've experienced and their impact on your health and the environment. Celebrate your progress and commit to continuing these sustainable practices.

Remember, every step towards sustainability and wellness is a victory worth celebrating. Keep moving forward and enjoy the journey!

Chapter 7

Social Wellness and Community Building

Imagine you're at a bustling coffee shop, surrounded by the chatter of friends catching up, colleagues discussing projects, and individuals deeply engrossed in books or laptops. This scene, vibrant with human connection, encapsulates the essence of social wellness—a fundamental aspect of holistic health that enriches our lives and buffers against the stresses of daily living. In this chapter, we delve into the art of building supportive relationships, a cornerstone of social wellness that not only enhances our emotional and mental well-being but also plays a critical role in our physical health and recovery processes.

Building Supportive Relationships

Understanding Support Systems

The value of a robust support system cannot be overstated. Psychologically, having a network of supportive relationships can significantly reduce stress, anxiety, and depression. Research consistently shows that individuals with strong social ties tend to live longer and experience better health outcomes. This phenomenon, often reflected in studies like those conducted by Julianne Holt-Lunstad at Brigham Young University, highlights that social connections can reduce mortality risk by up to 50%, underscoring the profound impact of our social environment on our longevity and vitality. These benefits are thought to arise because social support can buffer the physiological impacts of stress, and people within a supportive community often adopt healthier behaviors and feel a greater sense of purpose and belonging.

Cultivating Meaningful Connections

Developing these critical social ties means cultivating meaningful connections, both by deepening existing relationships and forming new ones. Active listening is a powerful tool in this endeavor. It involves fully concentrating on what is being said rather than passively hearing the message of the speaker. This practice helps build deeper, more empathetic connections, ensuring that your friends, family, and colleagues feel truly heard and valued. Shared activities also play a crucial role. Whether it's a weekly sports league, a book club, or a cooking class, engaging in regular communal activities can create a sense of camaraderie and commitment, strengthening bonds and providing regular social interaction which is key to building lasting relationships.

Navigating Challenges in Relationships

However, relationships aren't without their challenges. Conflicts and misunderstandings are inevitable, but the way we handle these situations can either strengthen or weaken our bonds. Effective communication skills are essential in navigating these waters. Techniques such as 'I' statements—expressing how you feel rather than accusing the other person—can foster understanding and prevent conflict escalation. Empathy also plays a crucial role; trying to see the situation from the other person's perspective can help resolve conflicts more amicably and maintain the strength of the relationship. Remember, the goal isn't to avoid all conflicts but to handle disagreements in ways that strengthen mutual understanding and respect.

Role of Support in Health Recovery

Support systems are particularly crucial during health challenges. Whether it's recovery from surgery, managing a chronic illness, or navigating mental health issues, having a network of supportive loved ones can significantly impact your recovery and ability to manage health conditions. They can offer practical help, like assisting with daily tasks or providing transportation to medical appointments, and emotional support, which can improve health outcomes. For instance, a study published in the *Journal of Clinical Oncology* found that breast cancer patients with robust social networks had significantly lower mortality rates and recurrence of cancer. These findings illuminate the powerful role that emotional support plays in the context of illness, highlighting how our social connections can quite literally be a lifeline during our most challenging moments.

Incorporating these aspects of building and maintaining supportive relationships into your life can transform your experience of the world. It enriches your emotional landscape, bolsters your mental resilience, and enhances your physical health. As you continue to weave these practices into the fabric of your daily life, you'll likely find that the quality of your relationships deepens, providing you with a stronger, more supportive network on which to lean, not just in times of need but every day. Engaging actively with this process of building and nurturing connections can turn each interaction into a meaningful exchange, enriching your life's tapestry with the threads of genuine relationships that support and uplift you through the complexities of life.

Communicating Needs and Boundaries

In the tapestry of daily interactions, whether with family, friends, or colleagues, the ability to effectively communicate your needs and set healthy boundaries is as crucial as any skill for maintaining your mental health and ensuring your relationships are both satisfying and supportive. Think about it this way: expressing your needs isn't just about getting what you want; it's about creating an environment where mutual understanding and respect flourish. This clarity helps prevent resentment and misunderstanding, which are often the root causes of relationship strain. For instance, clearly communicating your need for quiet time after work to decompress can help your family understand your actions and provide you with the space you need, thus avoiding feelings of neglect or irritation that might arise if you withdraw without explanation.

Setting boundaries is a natural extension of expressing your needs. It involves communicating to others what is acceptable and what is not, which helps manage their expectations and respects your limits. For instance, you might decide that you will not answer work calls during dinner time to ensure quality family time. It's important to convey these boundaries clearly and assertively, not apologetically. For example, you could say, "I value our team's hard work, but I won't be taking calls during dinner time to ensure I can recharge and be fully present for the next day's challenges." This kind of language not only sets a clear boundary but also communicates the value behind it, making it more likely to be respected.

Balancing self-care with caring for others is often a delicate dance, especially for those who naturally place others' needs before their own. The key here is to recognize that self-care is not selfish; rather, it's a prerequisite for effectively supporting others. Embracing the principle that one cannot give from an empty vessel is foundational to holistic wellness. Prioritizing your own needs ensures you are in the best position to support those you care about in a meaningful and sustained manner. This may involve dedicating moments for personal relaxation and rejuvenation before attending to the needs of others. Highlighting the significance of establishing personal boundaries, it's essential to understand that declining requests or asking for help as your energy depletes is not only acceptable but necessary. This practice not only protects your well-being but also sets a positive example, encouraging others to also treat their health with the same level of importance and care.

Dealing with pushback is often the most challenging aspect of setting boundaries. Not everyone will understand or respect your needs, and they may test your limits. It's crucial to stand firm in these situations and reiterate your boundaries with calm assertiveness. For example, if a family member repeatedly calls during your designated work hours, remind them of your availability with a gentle but firm reminder: "I understand you want to chat, which I love, but I need to focus on work during these hours. Can we schedule a call this evening instead?" If boundaries are continually disrespected, it might be necessary to seek external support, whether from other family members, friends, or a professional. This is not a failure but a proactive approach to maintaining your well-being and the health of your relationships.

Navigating the complexities of interpersonal dynamics through effective communication and boundary-setting is not just about avoiding conflict; it's about actively constructing a life that feels balanced, respectful, and fulfilling. As you improve in these areas, not only do your relationships deepen and become more satisfying, but your understanding of yourself and your needs becomes clearer. This clarity is empowering, enabling you to make choices that align more closely with your values and long-term well-being. As you continue to practice these skills, remember that each conversation is an opportunity to refine your approach and enhance your connections, making every interaction a stepping stone to a healthier, happier you.

Volunteering: The Health Benefits of Giving Back

When you lend a helping hand to others, the benefits extend far beyond the immediate impact of your actions. Engaging in volunteer activities can enrich your life in profound ways, boosting your emotional well-being and even enhancing your physical health. Think of it not just as giving back but as a key component of your holistic wellness strategy. Volunteering can infuse your life with a sense of purpose and fulfillment that is often hard to find in other pursuits. It's that heartwarming feeling you get when you see the direct impact of your efforts, whether you're helping to build a home, tutoring children, or planting trees in your community.

The emotional and psychological rewards of volunteering are immense. Engaging in altruistic activities can significantly boost your self-esteem and happiness. When you volunteer, you're often immersed in a supportive social environment that fosters positive interactions and teamwork. This social aspect can alleviate feelings of loneliness and depression by connecting you with others who share similar values and goals. Moreover, the act of helping others can give you a sense of purpose and satisfaction. A study from the London School of Economics found that people who volunteered were happier and felt they had better mental health compared to those who didn't. The researchers suggested that the personal rewards of volunteering are a vital component of the overall psychological benefits.

Volunteering also offers tangible physical health benefits. Regular volunteer work can significantly lower blood pressure, according to a study by Carnegie Mellon University, potentially reducing the risk of hypertension. This effect is thought to be connected to the stress-reducing properties of being helpful and working with others in a cooperative setting. Additionally, volunteering can increase longevity. A review of data from the Longitudinal Study of Aging found that those who volunteer have lower mortality rates than those who do not, even when controlling for physical health, age, and other factors. The physical activity involved in certain types of volunteer work can also contribute to better physical health, providing a low-stress workout environment that doesn't feel like exercise.

Finding the right volunteer opportunities is crucial in making sure that your efforts are as rewarding and impactful as possible. Start by identifying causes that resonate with your personal values and interests. Are you passionate about animal welfare, environmental conservation, or perhaps education? Once you've pinpointed areas you care about, look for organizations that work in those fields. Local nonprofits, religious groups, and community centers often have a variety of initiatives that could use help. When choosing a volunteering opportunity, consider how much time you can realistically commit. Some activities might require a regular weekly commitment, while others might be one-off events. By aligning your volunteering efforts with your personal values and time availability, you ensure that your experience is fulfilling and stress-free, allowing you to enjoy the emotional and physical benefits of your service fully.

Moreover, volunteering doesn't just benefit the individuals or communities being helped—it can also have a profound impact on the health of the broader community. Volunteers often bring energy and innovation to the organizations they work with, sparking improvements and inspiring others to contribute. This can lead to a more vibrant, active, and interconnected community. Furthermore, by addressing social issues and contributing to the common good, volunteering builds social capital, fostering stronger, more resilient communities that are better equipped to handle challenges and support their members. This interconnectedness of individual well-being and community health is a hallmark of the holistic approach to wellness, emphasizing that our health is deeply intertwined with the health of our social environment.

Group Fitness and Social Bonds

When you join a group fitness class or a sports league, you're signing up for more than just physical activity—you're stepping into a vibrant community of like-minded individuals who are there to motivate and uplift each other. The benefits of group exercise are manifold; not only does it enhance your physical fitness, but it also amplifies your motivation and enjoyment. Imagine the difference between jogging alone on a treadmill and participating in a lively group fitness class with upbeat music and enthusiastic companions. The energy in the room is contagious, pushing you to exert yourself more than you might have alone. This collective enthusiasm is a key element of group fitness that helps sustain participation over time, making your fitness journey a consistent and enjoyable one.

Moreover, group fitness provides a unique platform for social interaction and the formation of new friendships. Common goals and shared struggles naturally bring people together, creating a sense of camaraderie and mutual support. For instance, programs like CrossFit have a notorious reputation for fostering strong community bonds; members often celebrate each other's successes, whether it's achieving a personal best or completing a challenging workout. These social interactions are not limited to the time spent in the gym; many fitness groups organize social events outside of regular workout sessions, further strengthening the bonds between members. This social connectivity is crucial, as it can significantly enhance your commitment to a fitness regimen and make the overall experience more fulfilling.

The inclusivity of a fitness community is another critical factor that can greatly enhance your experience. An inclusive fitness community welcomes individuals of all skill levels and backgrounds, providing a supportive environment where everyone feels valued and capable of achieving their fitness goals. Creating such a community requires conscious effort and sensitivity from both instructors and participants. For example, fitness instructors can design programs that are adaptable to different fitness levels, ensuring that each participant can challenge themselves without feeling left behind. Participants, on the other hand, can foster an inclusive atmosphere by encouraging one another and respecting each individual's unique journey and pace.

A psychologically safe environment within fitness groups is essential for fostering a sense of security and belonging among members. Psychological safety means that members feel confident that they will not be exposed to discrimination, criticism, or any form of negative judgment based on their abilities or personal characteristics. This safety is crucial for allowing individuals to express themselves and engage fully without fear of embarrassment or rejection. For instance, a running club that celebrates each member's progress, regardless of pace, promotes a sense of achievement and belonging. Ensuring such an environment can encourage consistent participation and help individuals feel more connected to the group, enhancing both their physical and emotional well-being.

In essence, group fitness goes beyond physical health; it is a gateway to building stronger social connections and enhancing emotional health through community and inclusivity. As you continue to engage in these communal activities, you may find the social benefits to be just as rewarding as the physical ones. Each class, session, or event becomes an opportunity not just to enhance your fitness but to deepen your social interactions, broaden your support network, and enrich your overall quality of life.

Online Communities for Holistic Health Support

In today's digital age, the internet has revolutionized the way we seek and share health information. For anyone embarking on a journey toward holistic health, online communities—from dedicated forums and social media groups to specialized health apps—offer a wealth of resources right at your fingertips. These platforms can connect you with like-minded individuals across the globe, providing a space to share experiences, advice, and support. Imagine logging onto a forum and finding a thread discussing natural remedies for anxiety, or joining a Facebook group where members share their favorite vegetarian recipes. These interactions not only enrich your knowledge but also provide emotional support, making your wellness journey less isolating.

However, while these communities offer numerous benefits, they also come with their own set of challenges. The accessibility and anonymity of the internet can sometimes lead to the spread of misinformation. It's crucial to approach the information shared in these spaces with a critical eye. Verify the credibility of the sources and cross-check facts with reputable health websites or professionals. Additionally, the anonymity that makes it easy to share sensitive health issues also opens the door to potential cyberbullying or negative interactions. It's important to navigate these communities with caution, protecting your mental well-being by not engaging in or escalating online conflicts.

To foster positive interactions within these virtual spaces, it's essential to practice respectful communication and protect your privacy. Engage constructively by sharing your experiences and knowledge without making generalizations or giving unsolicited advice. Be mindful of the personal information you share, and set strict privacy settings on your accounts to control who can see your posts. By cultivating a respectful and cautious approach, you can make the most out of online communities without compromising your safety or peace of mind.

These online platforms can also serve as a bridge to real-world interactions, enhancing the tangible community support system. Many online groups organize local meetups or health-related events, providing an opportunity to connect face-to-face with those you've interacted with virtually. Participating in these events can deepen your connections and provide a sense of community that extends beyond the digital realm. Moreover, you can leverage these networks to initiate or participate in local wellness projects—such as starting a community garden or organizing a health fair—that benefit not just individual members but also the broader community. By integrating online interactions with real-world activities, you can enrich your holistic health journey with both global insights and local engagements, creating a well-rounded approach to wellness that leverages the best of both worlds.

Wellness Workshops and Local Events

Stepping into a local wellness workshop or attending a vibrant health fair isn't just about learning new things. It's about immersing yourself in a community that shares your interest in living better, healthier lives. Imagine the synergy of a group fitness challenge or the interactive learning at a seminar where every attendee is eager to improve their health and well-being. These local events offer invaluable opportunities to connect, learn, and grow in ways that daily routines seldom allow. They serve as essential platforms for exchanging ideas, encouraging each other, and even finding new inspiration to take your wellness journey further.

When you participate in these local gatherings, the educational benefits are immense. Seminars can introduce you to the latest health trends and evidence-based practices that you might not encounter online or in books. Health fairs often bring together a variety of practitioners, from nutritionists and personal trainers to holistic health experts, providing a broad spectrum of insights and services under one roof. Here, you can ask direct questions and receive immediate feedback, helping you better understand and navigate your health choices. Moreover, the social opportunities at these events are just as beneficial. Connecting with people who are also on their wellness paths can lead to new friendships and provide a sense of community that supports your own health goals. These interactions often create a motivational atmosphere that can reignite your passion for health and inspire you to pursue new practices or revitalize your existing routines.

Organizing community wellness activities can be a fulfilling endeavor that not only benefits your health but also enriches your local area. If you're inspired to bring wellness closer to home, start by identifying the needs and interests of your community. Perhaps a survey or informal conversations at local gatherings could provide insights into what topics or activities would garner the most interest. Once you've pinpointed these interests, reaching out to local health professionals, fitness instructors, or nutrition experts—who might be willing to participate or speak at your event—can add substantial value. Securing a venue is next, whether it's a community center, a park, or a school gym, depending on the size and nature of the event. Promoting your event through local businesses, schools, and social media will help attract a wider audience. Remember, the key to a successful event lies in good planning, clear communication, and a dash of creativity to make the experience both informative and enjoyable for all participants.

Incorporating both traditional and modern health practices into your events can cater to diverse preferences and increase the educational value of your gatherings. For instance, combining yoga sessions with workshops on the latest fitness technologies can appeal to different age groups and interests, providing a comprehensive overview of health and wellness. This approach not only broadens the appeal of your event but also encourages attendees to explore various facets of health and wellness that they may not have considered before.

Reflecting on successful events can provide valuable lessons and inspiration. Take, for example, a community that organized a "Health and Harmony" fair, which combined local artisan foods, yoga classes, and seminars on mental health. The event was a hit, drawing a large crowd and sparking interest in monthly follow-up meetings. Such successes underscore the positive impact that well-planned wellness events can have on a community's health and cohesion. They not only provide immediate health benefits and learning but also foster a collaborative spirit that can lead to sustained health initiatives within the community.

As we wrap up this chapter on community building through wellness workshops and local events, remember that these activities are more than just educational opportunities—they are a catalyst for creating healthier, more connected communities. By participating in or organizing these events, you contribute to a collective effort to enhance well-being on both a personal and community level. This chapter has equipped you with the knowledge to engage more deeply in your community's health landscape, whether by attending events, sharing your knowledge, or taking the lead in organizing. Each step you take builds towards a healthier, more vibrant community, reflecting the true essence of holistic wellness that extends beyond individual pursuits and nourishes the entire community.

> "Holistic wellness thrives on social wellness and community building, weaving a tapestry of interconnected lives that support and uplift each other."

Chapter 7 Wellness Plan: Social Wellness and Community Building

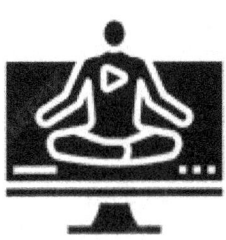

Activity: Cultivating Social Wellness

Take proactive steps to enhance your social wellness and build a supportive community around you. Reflect on each activity, document your experiences, and use music to enrich your journey.

Building Supportive Relationships:

◆ Identify three key people in your life who form your support system.

◆ Reach out to each person and express your appreciation.

◆ Plan a meaningful activity with one of them (e.g., a coffee date, a walk, or a shared hobby).

☆ ***Reflection:***

☆ *How did expressing appreciation affect your relationship?*

☆ What did you enjoy about the shared activity?

Communicating Needs and Boundaries:

◆ Identify a situation where you need to set a boundary or express a need.

◆ Use "I" statements to communicate this clearly and assertively.

☆ *Reflection:*

☆ How did the conversation go?

☆ What was the response, and how did you feel afterward?

Volunteering:

◆ Choose a local organization or cause to volunteer with.

◆ Dedicate at least one hour to volunteer work this week.

☆ *Reflection:*

☆ What activities did you engage in during your volunteering?

☆ How did volunteering make you feel emotionally and physically?

Group Fitness Participation:

◆ Join a group fitness class or a sports league.

◆ Attend at least one session.

☆ *Reflection:*

☆ Describe the atmosphere and energy of the group.

☆ How did participating in the group activity affect your motivation and enjoyment of exercise?

Engaging with Online Communities:
◆ Join an online health or wellness community (e.g., forum, Facebook group, health app).
◆ Participate in a discussion or share an experience.
☆ *Reflection:*
☆ What did you learn from the online community?
☆ How did it feel to connect with like-minded individuals?

Attending Wellness Workshops or Events:
◆ Find a local wellness workshop or health event to attend.
◆ Participate actively and network with other attendees.
☆ *Reflection:*
☆ What new information or skills did you learn?
☆ How did attending the event enhance your sense of community?

Organizing a Community Wellness Activity:
◆ Plan and organize a small wellness activity (e.g., a group walk, a healthy potluck, or a meditation session).
◆ Invite friends, family, or community members to join.
☆ *Reflection:*
☆ How did organizing and participating in the event feel?
☆ What was the feedback from the participants?

Music Suggestions:

◈ Energetic Playlist:

☆ *Curate a playlist of uplifting and energizing songs for group activities and fitness classes. Include tracks that foster a sense of community and motivation.*

◈ Calming Tunes for Reflection:

☆ *Create a playlist of soothing and reflective instrumental music for journaling and relaxation. Use these tunes to create a peaceful environment for your reflective activities.*

Acknowledge Your Effort:

Take a moment to celebrate the efforts you've made to build and strengthen your social wellness. Reflect on the positive changes and connections you've experienced. Recognize that each step you take towards building supportive relationships and engaging with your community contributes to your holistic health and well-being.

Remember, social wellness is a continuous journey. Each interaction and activity enriches your life, helping you create a network of support and connection that uplifts and sustains you through life's challenges and joys. Keep nurturing these relationships and communities, and enjoy the profound benefits they bring to your overall well-being.

Chapter 8

Adapting Wellness Into Your Unique Lifestyle

Tailoring Wellness Practices for Different Life Stages

Navigating through life's stages can sometimes feel like trying to stitch a quilt from different fabrics, each piece representing a different phase with its unique texture and color. From the vibrant, fast-paced days of youth, through the transformative years of midlife, to the reflective season of seniority, each stage demands different wellness strategies. Understanding and adapting these strategies to align with your life phase not only enhances your well-being but also ensures that your wellness journey is rich, fulfilling, and, most importantly, effective.

Identifying Needs by Life Stage

The beauty of life lies in its dynamism and diversity—qualities that are mirrored in our evolving wellness needs. During the energetic years of youth and early adulthood, the focus often leans towards maintaining high energy levels and managing stress, particularly from career building and social dynamics. As you transition into midlife, the narrative shifts slightly towards maintaining optimum physical health, managing the stress that comes with life's peak responsibilities, and preparing for a healthy older age. This preparation might involve more focused preventive health measures such as regular screenings and adopting a heart-healthy diet. When you step into the golden years, the focus pivots towards preserving mobility, cognitive function, and social engagement. Each stage builds upon the previous, and understanding this progression can help you tailor your wellness practices to better meet your changing needs.

Youth and Wellness

For young adults, integrating wellness amidst the whirlwind of establishing careers and navigating social landscapes can be daunting. Energy management becomes crucial. Simple practices like maintaining a balanced diet rich in whole foods can provide sustained energy throughout the day. Incorporating physical activities that align with your interests—be it yoga, cycling, or team sports—can significantly boost your physical and mental health. However, mental wellness should not be overlooked. Techniques such as mindfulness meditation or journaling can be powerful tools for managing stress and anxiety, fostering a sense of inner peace that supports your overall well-being.

Midlife Wellness Strategies

As you move into midlife, maintaining your physical health becomes increasingly important. This stage often involves juggling multiple roles—professional, parent, spouse, caregiver—all of which can take a toll on your health if not managed well. Stress management is key. Regular physical activity, such as brisk walking or swimming, can help mitigate stress while also combating the metabolic slowdown associated with aging. Additionally, this is a critical time to invest in preventive health measures. Regular health screenings, such as blood pressure checks, cholesterol levels, and diabetes screenings, become vital. These proactive steps can help you catch potential health issues early, making them easier to manage or even reverse.

Senior Health Focus

In the later years of life, the emphasis shifts towards maintaining mobility, cognitive function, and social connections. Adapting exercises to accommodate any physical limitations is crucial. Low-impact activities like tai chi, water aerobics, or chair yoga can be beneficial. These activities not only help maintain muscle strength and flexibility but also enhance balance, reducing the risk of falls. Nutrition also plays a pivotal role; diets rich in omega-3 fatty acids, antioxidants, and soluble fibers can support cognitive function and overall health. Social engagement, often overlooked, is critical during this stage. Participating in community activities or volunteer work can provide both mental stimulation and a sense of purpose, enriching your later years with joy and connectivity.

Adapting your wellness routine to suit your current life stage is not just about adding or modifying activities; it's about creating a harmonious blend of practices that resonate with your body's needs and your life's demands. This personalized approach ensures that your wellness journey is not only about longevity but about enhancing the quality of life at every stage. As you transition through life's different seasons, keep in mind that each stage offers unique opportunities for growth and health, and with the right strategies, you can thrive through them all.

Overcoming the Guilt of Self-Care

In today's fast-paced society, taking a moment for oneself can sometimes feel like a luxury or, worse, a mark of selfishness. This is especially true for those who juggle multiple roles—parents, caregivers, professionals—who often find themselves postponing their own needs to cater to others'. The stigma associated with self-care is rooted deeply in cultural narratives that praise tirelessness and criticize self-focus. However, dismantling these perceptions is crucial, not only for your well-being but also for maintaining your ability to care for others effectively.

Addressing the stigma involves reshaping how we perceive self-care, starting with recognizing that it is an absolute necessity, not a luxury. Psychological insights tell us that neglecting self-care can lead to burnout—a state of emotional, physical, and mental exhaustion caused by prolonged stress. This not only diminishes your ability to perform daily tasks but also affects your health and relationships negatively. It's essential to challenge the old paradigms that associate self-care with guilt. Instead, view it as a preventive strategy that keeps you healthy and energized, thus enabling you to be more present and supportive in the lives of those you care about.

Balancing self-care with responsibilities may seem like a daunting task, but it can be managed with the right strategies. Effective time management is key. Start by assessing how you currently spend your time. Identify activities that do not add value or joy to your life. Could these be minimized or eliminated? Next, prioritize tasks using the Eisenhower Box technique, which helps you decide on and prioritize tasks by urgency and importance, focusing on what truly needs your attention. Additionally, setting clear boundaries is crucial; it's okay to say no or delegate tasks to ensure you're not over-committing yourself. This not only helps prevent burnout but also frees up time to engage in rejuvenating activities that enhance your well-being.

Reinforcing the idea that self-care is a necessity involves a shift in mindset and culture within families, workplaces, and communities. It's about understanding that taking care of your health—physical, mental, and emotional—is fundamental to living a full and capable life. Research consistently shows that well-rested, mentally healthy individuals perform better at work and maintain healthier relationships. Encouraging a culture where taking time for mental health is normalized can lead to more productive and happy individuals. For instance, companies that implement policies supporting mental health days and encourage regular breaks see improved employee satisfaction and productivity.

To illustrate the positive effects of self-care, let's look at Maria, a healthcare professional and mother. Initially overwhelmed by her responsibilities, Maria attended a work-life balance workshop and learned to set firm boundaries and allocate time for hobbies. This not only boosted her mental health but also enhanced her engagement and productivity both at home and at work. Similarly, John, a senior software developer, incorporated short mindfulness walks into his workday, experiencing increased focus and reduced stress. These instances demonstrate how integrating self-care strategies can significantly improve personal and professional well-being, emphasizing its importance and effectiveness.

Integrating Wellness into the Workday

When you think about your workday, it's often a balancing act between productivity and well-being. But what if you could integrate both seamlessly? Workplace wellness programs are more than just a corporate trend; they are a pivot toward a healthier, more engaged workforce. Participating in or even initiating these programs can transform your work environment into a space that supports holistic health, encompassing exercise, mindfulness, and healthy eating initiatives. Imagine the boost in morale and reduction in stress when employees have access to structured wellness activities right at their workplace. These programs could range from organized group workouts to scheduled mindfulness sessions, all designed to reduce stress and promote health without stepping out of the office.

Now, let's talk about incorporating these wellness practices directly into your daily routine. Desk exercises and proper ergonomics play a crucial role here. It's easy to underestimate the strain that prolonged sitting can have on your body. Integrating simple exercises into your workday can significantly alleviate this. For instance, every couple of hours, you could perform stretches specifically designed for office environments—like neck rolls and wrist stretches—or even maintain a mini stepper under your desk for a quick cardio session. Pairing these physical activities with an ergonomic workstation setup—ensuring that your monitor is at eye level and your chair supports your lower back—can drastically reduce the risk of strain and injury, promoting better physical health and greater comfort throughout your workday.

Mental resets are equally important. They help maintain focus and reduce stress, key components in enhancing work performance and overall well-being. Simple practices like taking short meditative breaks or engaging in walking meetings can provide these mental refreshes. Imagine replacing a traditional conference room meeting with a walking meeting outside. This not only fosters a dynamic discussion but also incorporates physical activity into your agenda, hitting two birds with one stone. Additionally, mindfulness sessions, even if brief, can be incorporated throughout the day to help clear the mind and relieve stress. Techniques such as focused breathing or visualization can be done right at your desk and are effective methods for recalibrating your mental state, keeping you sharp and centered.

Balancing work and personal life is paramount, and it often starts in the workplace. Setting clear boundaries is essential; it's important to communicate effectively with your team about your availability and work hours to ensure you have time to recharge after work. Effective stress management also plays a crucial role. This could involve setting realistic daily goals, which helps in managing expectations and reducing the urge to overextend yourself. Furthermore, encouraging a culture that prioritizes wellness can lead to more sustainable work practices, including recognizing the signs of burnout and encouraging regular breaks among team members. These strategies not only enhance individual well-being but also foster a supportive and productive work environment.

Incorporating these elements into your workday isn't just about personal health; it's about fostering a workplace culture that values and actively promotes wellness. By integrating physical exercises, ergonomic solutions, mental health practices, and a well-balanced approach to work and life, you can create a more productive, enjoyable, and healthy work environment. This holistic approach not only benefits individual employees but also contributes to a more vibrant, energetic, and healthy workplace culture.

The Role of Personal Development in Wellness

Exploring the realms of personal development is akin to planting a garden of diverse experiences—it nurtures your mind, enriches your emotions, and cultivates a healthier, more resilient you. From learning a new language to picking up a musical instrument, or diving into a creative hobby like painting, each new skill or hobby you acquire doesn't just fill your time—it enhances your cognitive abilities, boosts your emotional well-being, and integrates seamlessly with your holistic health goals. This fusion of lifelong learning and wellness is not just about adding activities to your busy schedule; it's about enriching your life's tapestry with vibrant threads of growth and satisfaction.

Lifelong Learning and Wellness

The connection between personal development and wellness is profound. Engaging in continuous learning has been shown to improve brain function, enhance emotional regulation, and increase life satisfaction. When you challenge your brain with new skills, you're essentially strength-training it, making it stronger and more adaptable. This mental agility can translate into better problem-solving skills, a sharper memory, and delayed cognitive decline as you age. Moreover, the joy and satisfaction derived from mastering a new skill can be a significant mood booster, reducing stress and contributing to your overall happiness.

Personal development also fosters a sense of accomplishment and self-efficacy. When you learn to play a new instrument, for instance, not only do you enjoy the music you create, but you also build confidence in your ability to tackle new challenges. This confidence can permeate other areas of your life, improving your overall approach to challenges and setbacks. Additionally, hobbies and continuous learning often provide opportunities for social interaction, whether through classes, clubs, or online communities. These social connections are vital for emotional health, offering support, inspiration, and camaraderie.

Setting Personal Growth Goals

When integrating personal development into your wellness strategy, setting clear, achievable goals is crucial. These goals should be specific, measurable, achievable, relevant, and time-bound (SMART). For instance, if you're interested in photography, a SMART goal could be, "Enroll in an introductory photography course at the community center and complete it by the end of the quarter." This goal is specific (take a course), measurable (complete the course), achievable (introductory level), relevant (interest in photography), and time-bound (by the end of the quarter).

Setting personal growth goals helps maintain your focus and makes the process of learning new skills more structured and rewarding. It also allows you to track your progress, which can be incredibly motivating. Reflect on your interests and how they align with your long-term wellness goals. For example, if stress reduction is a priority, you might choose activities known for their calming effects, like yoga or knitting. Alternatively, if enhancing cognitive function is your goal, learning a new language or instrument can be particularly beneficial.

Integrating Personal and Professional Growth

Balancing personal interests with professional development can enhance both your career and personal life. For many, professional growth is closely linked to personal satisfaction. However, it's important to find harmony between the two, ensuring that one does not overshadow the other. For instance, if you're a marketing professional interested in graphic design, taking a course in this field can enrich your skill set, making your work more fulfilling and opening up new career opportunities. Similarly, developing skills like public speaking or project management can boost your confidence and performance in personal endeavors like community volunteering or running a club.

Integrating personal and professional development involves continuous reflection and adjustment. It's about understanding how the skills you acquire in one area can benefit the other. This holistic approach not only leads to a more satisfying career but also enriches your personal life, making you a more well-rounded, content, and capable individual.

Resources for Personal Development

Fortunately, the resources available for personal development are vast and varied. Books, online courses, workshops, and podcasts can provide the guidance and inspiration you need to embark on your learning journey. Websites like Coursera or Udemy offer a plethora of courses in virtually any field imaginable, from science and technology to art and music. Local community centers, libraries, and colleges frequently provide classes and workshops that can offer both learning opportunities and a chance to connect with like-minded individuals.

Choosing resources that fit your learning style, schedule, and budget is key. For those with tight schedules, podcasts or audiobooks can be a perfect fit, offering the flexibility to learn while commuting or during other routine activities. For hands-on learners, workshops or physical classes provide immediate feedback and engagement that can be crucial for mastering new skills. Whatever resources you choose, ensure they align with your goals and provide the level of depth and engagement you need to stay motivated and inspired on your path to personal and professional fulfillment.

By weaving personal development into the fabric of your wellness strategy, you're not just learning new things; you're enhancing your overall quality of life, and building a resilient, capable, and satisfied self. Whether through developing new skills, setting growth-oriented goals, balancing personal and professional development, or utilizing diverse resources, the journey of personal development is a fulfilling path that promotes a healthier, happier you.

Keeping Wellness Engaging and New

Maintaining an engaging and fresh approach to your wellness routine is much like keeping a garden; it requires variety, attention to seasonal shifts, and the integration of new tools and technologies to thrive. Let's explore how you can invigorate your fitness and nutrition regimen, weave social wellness activities into your routine, adapt your practices to align with the changing seasons and harness innovative wellness technologies to keep your wellness journey lively and enjoyable.

Variety in Fitness and Nutrition

Sticking to the same workout routine or meal plan can quickly become tedious, leading to a plateau not just in your physical progress but in your enthusiasm as well. Injecting variety into your fitness and nutrition regimen can rekindle your interest and boost your motivation. Consider incorporating new forms of exercise into your routine. If you've always been a runner, why not try a dance class or take up swimming? Each sport engages different muscle groups and can be refreshing mentally and physically. Similarly, exploring new dietary changes can revitalize your interest in healthy eating. Enroll in a cooking class to master a cuisine you're unfamiliar with, or challenge yourself to a 'vegetable of the week' club where you try new or unusual vegetables in your meals. These changes keep your diet exciting and can lead to new discoveries about foods and cooking techniques that benefit your health.

Social Wellness Activities

Incorporating a social element into your wellness practices can dramatically enhance your engagement and commitment. Humans are inherently social beings, and we thrive on connection. Participating in group activities, whether joining a hiking club, enrolling in a group meditation class, or attending a fitness boot camp, provides not only companionship but also the motivation for shared goals. These activities allow you to connect with others who are on similar wellness paths, offering mutual encouragement and making the activities more enjoyable. The camaraderie developed in these social settings can be a powerful motivator, turning the solitary pursuit of wellness into a shared endeavor that brings joy and enhanced commitment to your health goals.

Seasonal Wellness Changes

Just as nature cycles through seasons, your wellness routine can benefit from adjustments that align with seasonal changes. This keeps your routine aligned with the natural world and prevents monotony from creeping into your activities. During the warmer months, take advantage of the weather to engage in outdoor activities such as cycling, outdoor yoga, or beach volleyball. As the weather cools, transition to indoor activities like joining a gym, trying indoor rock climbing, or swimming in an indoor pool. Seasonal changes can also be reflected in your diet; summer might focus on salads and smoothies while winter shifts to warm soups and roasted vegetables. Embracing the rhythm of the seasons keeps your activities fresh and attuned to the natural environment, enhancing your physical and mental well-being.

Innovative Wellness Tools and Tech

The ever-evolving landscape of technology offers new avenues to enhance your wellness practices. From fitness trackers that monitor your physical activity and sleep patterns to apps that provide guided meditation sessions, technology can be a valuable ally in your wellness journey. Wearable devices can help you stay on track with your fitness goals by providing real-time data on your performance and progress. Similarly, virtual reality experiences can offer immersive meditation or yoga sessions that transport you to calming environments, enhancing your relaxation and mindfulness practices. Apps that track your dietary intake and offer nutritious recipes can make maintaining a healthy diet easier and more enjoyable. By integrating these technological tools into your wellness regimen, you can add an element of fun and discovery, keeping your routine engaging and tailored to your evolving needs.

As you continue to explore these strategies, remember that the key to a vibrant wellness journey lies in staying curious and open to new experiences. Whether through trying new physical activities, connecting with others, adapting to the seasons, or integrating cutting-edge technology, there are endless opportunities to infuse excitement and novelty into your path to health and well-being. Keep exploring, keep experimenting, and keep enjoying every step of your wellness adventure.

Reviewing and Renewing Your Wellness Goals Annually

Reflecting on your wellness journey once a year isn't just about checking boxes; it's a crucial practice that helps align your actions with your evolving life circumstances and personal aspirations. It's like pausing on a hike to ensure you're still on the right path and making adjustments to reach the summit efficiently. This annual review is your opportunity to look back on what you've achieved, learn from what didn't go as planned, and set new goals that ignite your motivation. It's about maintaining a dynamic approach to your wellness, ensuring that your strategies remain relevant and motivating as your life changes.

Importance of Regular Reviews

Conducting regular reviews of your wellness goals serves multiple purposes. It allows you to see the progress you've made, which can be incredibly motivating. Reflecting on the successes, even the small ones, can fuel your desire to continue. More importantly, this review process helps you identify strategies that may no longer be effective or relevant. Life changes—perhaps you've moved to a new city, changed jobs, or experienced significant changes in your personal life—these shifts can all impact your wellness routine. By taking the time to assess your goals annually, you can make informed decisions about what to continue, what to stop, and what new goals you might want to pursue. This adaptability is key to maintaining a wellness routine that fits your current lifestyle and continues to bring you joy and health.

Setting SMART Goals

To ensure your wellness goals are clear and reachable, each one should be SMART—Specific, Measurable, Achievable, Relevant, and Time-bound. This framework not only guides your planning process but also enhances the likelihood of achieving your goals. For instance, instead of setting a vague goal like "get fit," a SMART goal would be "attend three yoga classes per week for the next three months." This goal is specific (attend yoga classes), measurable (three times a week), achievable (a realistic number of classes per week), relevant (contributes to your fitness), and time-bound (for the next three months). Using this structured approach in your annual planning helps turn abstract aspirations into actionable steps, making it easier to track progress and make adjustments as needed.

Celebrating Achievements and Learning from Setbacks

Each review is a chance to celebrate your successes and learn from the setbacks. When assessing your past year, take note of the achievements, no matter how small. Did you stick to your goal of meditating each morning? Did you make dietary changes that improved your health? Celebrating these victories reinforces your efforts and boosts your confidence. Likewise, it's important to reflect on the goals you didn't meet. Understanding why certain goals were not achieved can provide valuable insights. Was the goal too ambitious? Did unforeseen circumstances interfere? Analyzing these setbacks helps you learn and grow, ensuring that your future goals are more aligned with your capabilities and life situation.

Planning for Upcoming Years

Looking forward involves anticipating changes in your life that might impact your wellness routine. Maybe you're approaching a significant birthday, anticipating career changes, or your children are growing older, and your daily schedule will be different. These life events can significantly impact your wellness needs and the time you have available for wellness activities. By planning with these changes in mind, you can adapt your goals so that they continue to be relevant and achievable. For example, if you know a busy work period is approaching, you might focus on stress management techniques rather than intensive physical fitness goals. Planning for the future with foresight allows you to maintain continuity in your wellness journey, adapting smoothly to life's ebbs and flows.

As you wrap up your annual wellness review, take a moment to appreciate the journey you've been on. The insights you gain from this reflective process are invaluable, helping you to sculpt a wellness plan that not only meets your needs but also sparks joy and fulfillment in your everyday life. Looking ahead, you're equipped not just with goals, but with a deeper understanding of how to live well, no matter what life throws your way. Moving forward, you'll continue to refine, adjust, and thrive, carrying with you the lessons learned and the successes celebrated.

<u>Next Steps</u>

As we close this chapter on reviewing and renewing your wellness goals, remember that this process is an integral part of living a mindful, healthy life. It's about taking control of your well-being, celebrating your progress, and learning from every experience. Up next, we'll explore how to integrate these principles into broader aspects of your life, ensuring that wellness remains a joyful and rewarding part of your everyday existence.

"Embracing wellness within your unique lifestyle transforms health into a personal journey, harmonizing your well-being with your individual needs and aspirations."

Chapter 8 Wellness Plan: Adapting Wellness Into Your Unique Lifestyle

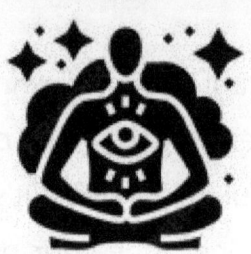

Activity: Annual Wellness Goals Review

Objective: Reflect on your past year's wellness journey, celebrate achievements, learn from setbacks, and set new goals for the upcoming year.

Step 1: Reflect on Achievements

★ List 3 wellness goals you achieved this year. Describe how you feel about these achievements.

Music Suggestion: "Happy" by Pharrell Williams

Step 2: Learn from Setbacks

★ Identify 2 wellness goals you didn't achieve. Reflect on the reasons why and what you learned from these experiences.

Music Suggestion: "Fix You" by Coldplay

Step 3: Set New SMART Goals

★ Write down 3 new wellness goals for the upcoming year. Ensure they are Specific, Measurable, Achievable, Relevant, and Time-bound (SMART).

Music Suggestion: "Eye of the Tiger" by Survivor

Step 4: Plan for Future Changes

★ Note any anticipated changes in your life (e.g., job change, moving) and how they might impact your wellness routine. Plan adjustments accordingly.

Music Suggestion: "Here Comes the Sun" by The Beatles

Step 5: Celebrate and Motivate

★ Write a short paragraph on how you will celebrate your achievements and stay motivated throughout the next year.

Music Suggestion: "Don't Stop Believin'" by Journey

End with Reflection

★ Spend 5 minutes reflecting on your wellness journey while listening to "What a Wonderful World" by Louis Armstrong.

Worksheet Summary:

- **Reflect on Achievements:** Celebrate your successes.

- **Learn from Setbacks:** Understand and grow from

what didn't work.

- **Set New SMART Goals:** Define clear, actionable goals.

- **Plan for Changes:** Prepare for future life events.

- **Celebrate and Motivate:** Keep your journey joyful and inspiring.

Chapter 9

Bonus Chapter: Ask the Wellness Coach

Real Questions. Practical Answers. No Judgment.

You asked, we answered. Here are some of the most common wellness questions I've received—from people just like you who are trying to live better without the overwhelm. Let's bust some myths, keep it real, and help you move forward with confidence.

Q: "Do I have to be vegetarian or vegan to be healthy?"

A: Not at all! While plant-based diets have great benefits, holistic wellness is about balance, not labels. You can be an omnivore and still make mindful choices—like eating more whole foods, cutting down on processed stuff, and being intentional with what goes on your plate.

Q: "I'm so busy. How do I even start a wellness plan?"

A: Start *tiny*. One glass of water when you wake up. Five minutes of deep breathing. A walk during your lunch break. You don't need an hour-long morning routine to feel better—you just need *consistency*, not perfection. Stack simple habits and build from there.

Q: "What's the best time of day to meditate or exercise?"

A: The best time is when *you'll actually do it*. Morning routines get a lot of hype, but if you're not a morning person, it's okay. Wellness isn't a race—it's a rhythm. Whether it's sunrise stretches or midnight journaling, the "right" time is the time that fits *your* life.

Q: "Is it okay to skip a day or fall off track?"

A: 100% yes. Life isn't a straight line, and your wellness journey won't be either. Progress isn't ruined by one skipped workout or a weekend of takeout. What matters is that you get back on track with *compassion*, not guilt. You're human. You're allowed to be flexible.

Q: "How do I deal with negative self-talk?"

A: Name it. Call it out. Replace it. Try saying:
- "This is a tough moment, but I'm doing my best."
- "I choose progress, not perfection."
- "I'm worthy of feeling well."
  Your mind believes what you repeat. Choose to be kind to yourself.

Q: "Is holistic wellness expensive?"

A: It doesn't have to be! Many wellness practices are *free*: walking, breathing, journaling, sleeping better, drinking water. Sure, there are fancy products out there, but the foundation of true wellness is simple, sustainable, and accessible to all.

Q: "Where do I go from here?"

A: Use this book as your starting point. Revisit the parts that resonated. Pick *one* area—like nutrition, movement, or mindset—and take a small, doable step today. Wellness isn't a destination—it's a plan you can live with, one intentional choice at a time.

Q: "I want to eat healthy, but I hate cooking. Help?"

A: You don't have to be a chef to eat well. Think lazy-gourmet: rotisserie chicken + salad kit, smoothie packs, pre-chopped veggies. Batch cooking on Sundays can be a game-changer. Or go for no-cook options—Greek yogurt, nuts, fruit, overnight oats. Eating healthy doesn't have to mean hours in the kitchen.

Q: "What if my family isn't on board with my wellness goals?"

A: Focus on your lane. Be the inspiration, not the enforcer. Invite them in with curiosity: "Want to try this smoothie?" or "Join me for a walk?" Lead by example. Even small shifts in your energy can influence those around you more than lectures ever will.

Q: "How do I stay consistent when I keep losing motivation?"

A: Motivation is fickle. Build systems instead. Put your yoga mat where you can see it. Schedule walks like meetings. Use apps, reminders, playlists—whatever works. When motivation fades (and it will), your habits will carry you forward.

Q: "What's something I can do right now to feel better instantly?"

A: Breathe. Inhale for 4, hold for 4, exhale for 6. Do it 3 times. You've just calmed your nervous system. Then, get up and stretch, drink some water, or step outside. Tiny shifts = big impact when done consistently.

Q: "Can I include wine or dessert in a holistic lifestyle?"

A: Absolutely. Deprivation isn't wellness—*balance* is. Enjoy your glass of wine or a slice of cake mindfully and without guilt. The key is presence. Savor the moment, and let joy be part of your plan.

Q: "How do I know if I'm making progress?"

A: Progress isn't just weight or numbers. Ask yourself:
- Am I sleeping better?
- Do I feel calmer or more energized?
- Am I making better choices more often than not? Progress is personal. Celebrate the wins that don't show up on the scale.

Q: "What if I don't like gyms or traditional workouts?"

A: Great! Movement comes in many forms: dancing in your room, walking your dog, yoga on YouTube, biking, gardening, swimming, even cleaning with music on full blast. The best workout is the one you'll *actually enjoy*.

Q: "How do I unplug when I feel addicted to my phone?"

A: Try a mini digital detox:
- No screens during meals.
- Phone-free mornings for 30 minutes.
- Use "Do Not Disturb" mode after a certain time. Replace scrolling with something soothing—reading, journaling, stretching, or just sitting with a cup of tea.

Q: "Is holistic wellness spiritual or religious?"

A: It can be—but it doesn't have to be. Some find spiritual growth through prayer or meditation, others through nature, creativity, or service. Holistic wellness simply means you honor your whole self—body, mind, and spirit—whatever that means *to you*.

Q: "What if I mess up... again?"

A: You're not starting over. You're *starting from experience*. Wellness isn't about flawless execution. It's about showing up for yourself with grace, again and again. Forgive yourself. Then take the next best step.

Chapter 10

Conclusion

As we draw the curtains on this enriching journey through the realms of holistic wellness, let's take a moment to reflect on the path we've traveled together. From exploring the foundational aspects of holistic health to diving into practical nutrition, engaging in physical fitness, nurturing our mental and emotional well-being, and expanding into the spiritual and environmental dimensions of health, we've covered a vast landscape of knowledge and practices. Each chapter was designed not just to inform but to transform—encouraging you to weave these insights into the fabric of your daily life.

One of the most profound lessons we've embraced is the deep interconnectedness of our wellness dimensions. Your physical health influences your mental state, your emotional balance feeds into your spiritual well-being, and your environment impacts them all. This intricate web of connections underscores why a holistic approach is not just beneficial but essential for anyone seeking a truly balanced and healthy life.

Yet, as we've discovered, there is no universal blueprint for achieving wellness. Each of you brings your unique set of circumstances, needs, and preferences to the table. This diversity is not a challenge but a beautiful opportunity to tailor the principles we've discussed to craft a personal wellness journey that resonates deeply with your individual lifestyle and goals.

Embracing the spirit of continuous learning and adaptation is crucial as you forge ahead. The landscape of health and wellness is ever-evolving, with new insights, techniques, and technologies emerging regularly. Stay curious, remain flexible, and be willing to adjust your strategies as you grow and as new information becomes available. This openness will not only enhance your journey but also ensure it remains vibrant and fulfilling.

Now, I urge you to take that first, brave step toward integrating these holistic practices into your daily routine. Whether it's setting aside a few minutes each day for mindfulness, experimenting with nutritious recipes, or connecting with nature, each small step is a leap towards a fuller, more vibrant life.

Share your journey with others. There is immense power in community and shared experiences. By connecting with others who are also walking this path, you'll find not just companionship but also mutual inspiration and support. Together, you can celebrate successes, navigate challenges, and perhaps even inspire others to join in this beautiful pursuit of wellness.

Remember, the ultimate goal of embracing holistic wellness is to enrich your life, not just to extend it. It's about growing, learning, and thriving, reaching towards your fullest potential in all aspects of life. As you reflect on your personal wellness goals, think about what truly matters to you. Set intentions that are not just achievable but also deeply fulfilling.

Thank you sincerely for joining me on this journey. Your commitment to exploring and adopting a holistic approach to wellness is not just a gift to yourself but to those around you, as you become a beacon of health, balance, and vitality. Here's to moving forward with grace, strength, and joy on your continuous path to wellness. May you find the balance you seek, and may your life be all the richer for it. Cheers to good health, profound growth, and a vibrant life ahead!

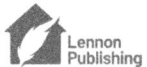

Thank you for reading *The Ultimate Holistic Essentials: A Complete Wellness and Fitness Collection with Mindfulness and Healthy Diet for Everyday Living.*

If this collection helped you build better habits, feel more balanced, or inspired new routines, we'd truly appreciate your feedback. Your review helps more readers discover practical ways to bring mindfulness and fitness into their daily lives.

You can scan the QR code or visit our review page to share your thoughts. It only takes a moment but makes a lasting difference for independent publishers like us.

References

- AMA Journal of Ethics. (2008, March). Holistic medicine and Western medical tradition. https://journalofethics.ama-assn.org/article/holistic-medicine-and-western-medical-tradition/2008-03

- American Psychological Association. (n.d.). How stress affects your health. https://www.apa.org/topics/stress/health

- ATLWell. (n.d.). Gratitude journaling: A daily practice for mental health. https://www.atlwell.com/blog/gratitude-journaling

- Bija Bennet. (n.d.). 4 steps to creating a personal ritual. https://www.bijab.com/wellness-blog/how-to-create-a-personal-ritual/

- Cleveland Clinic. (n.d.). Music therapy: Types & benefits. https://my.clevelandclinic.org/health/treatments/8817-music-therapy

- Fitness Project. (n.d.). 8 quick and effective workouts for busy professionals. https://fitnessproject.us/blog/8-quick-and-effective-workouts-for-busy-professionals/

- Food Network. (n.d.). Water: How much should you drink every day? https://www.foodnetwork.com/recipes/photos/our-best-healthy-recipes-for-kids-and-families

- Global Wellness Summit. (n.d.). 12 wellness trends for 2023. https://www.globalwellnesssummit.com/press/press-releases/12-wellness-trends-for-2023/

- Greenleaf Communities. (n.d.). The many benefits of community gardens. https://www.greenleafcommunities.org/the-many-benefits-of-community-gardens/

- Harvard Health. (n.d.). Foods linked to better brainpower. https://thegirlonbloor.com/52-healthy-quick-easy-dinner-ideas-for-busy-weeknights/

- Healthline. (n.d.). 9 types of meditation: Which one is right for you? https://www.healthline.com/health/mental-health/types-of-meditation#:~:text=Not%20all%20meditation%20styles%20are,meditation%20author%20and%20holistic%20nutritionist.

- IHRSA. (n.d.). Creating an inclusive fitness club and sector. https://www.ihrsa.org/publications/creating-an-inclusive-fitness-club-and-sector-an-ihrsa-e-book/

- Mayo Clinic. (n.d.). Mindfulness exercises. https://www.mayoclinic.org/healthy-lifestyle/consumer-health/in-depth/mindfulness-exercises/art-20046356

- Mind. (n.d.). How nature benefits mental health. https://www.mind.org.uk/information-support/tips-for-everyday-living/nature-and-mental-health/how-nature-benefits-mental-health/

- Performance Health. (n.d.). 20 family fitness ideas beyond the gym. https://www.performancehealth.com/articles/20-family-fitness-ideas-beyond-the-gym/

- Psychological Healthcare. (n.d.). How life stages may affect your mental health. https://www.psychologicalhealthcare.com.au/blog/life-stages-mental-health/

- PubMed Central. (n.d.). Exploring the effects of volunteering on social, mental, and physical health. https://www.ncbi.nlm.nih.gov/pmc/articles/PMC10159229/

- PubMed Central. (n.d.). Foods that fight inflammation. https://www.ncbi.nlm.nih.gov/pmc/articles/PM

C4780815/

- PubMed Central. (n.d.). How the glycemic index can impact your mental health. https://www.ncbi.nlm.nih.gov/pmc/articles/PMC2805706/

- PubMed Central. (n.d.). Plant-based dietary patterns for human and planetary health. https://www.ncbi.nlm.nih.gov/pmc/articles/PMC9024616/

- PubMed Central. (n.d.). Sense of community and mental health: A cross-sectional analysis. https://www.ncbi.nlm.nih.gov/pmc/articles/PMC10314672/

- Self. (n.d.). 53 bodyweight exercises you can do at home. https://www.self.com/gallery/bodyweight-exercises-you-can-do-at-home

- Today. (n.d.). Walking benefits: The physical and mental benefits of walks. https://www.today.com/health/physical-mental-benefits-walking-t207904

- University of Georgia. (n.d.). 10 strategies for better time management. https://extension.uga.edu/publications/detail.html?number=C1042&title=time-management-10-strategies-for-better-time-management

- U.S. Department of Energy. (n.d.). Reducing electricity

use and costs. https://www.energy.gov/energysaver/reducing-electricity-use-and-costs

- Verywell Mind. (2024). 10 best mental health and therapy apps of 2024. https://www.verywellmind.com/best-mental-health-apps-4692902

- WebMD. (n.d.). What is holistic medicine and how does it work? https://www.webmd.com/balance/what-is-holistic-medicine

HOLISTIC LIVING *for* FITNESS

A Mindful Approach to Workouts, Meal Planning, and Lasting Weight Loss in a Hectic World

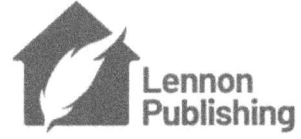

Contents

Introduction	198
1. Embracing the Mind-Body Connection	201
2. Mindful Nutrition Essentials	225
3. Personalized Fitness for Every Lifestyle	247
4. Creating Lasting Habits	269
5. Mindful Living and Stress Management	287
6. Ethical and Environmental Considerations	303
7. Interactive Journaling for Self-Discovery	321
8. Enhancing Your Wellness Journey with Technology	340
9. Conclusion	359
Extended Edition: Travel-Friendly Workouts	362
Bonus Chapter: Fitness Myths Debunked Separating Fact from Fiction	369
References	378

Introduction

You're running late for work, juggling a phone call and a half-eaten sandwich, and the idea of fitting in a workout today seems laughable. Sound familiar? For many of us, life feels like a never-ending race against the clock. We're trying to balance our careers, families, and social lives, often at the expense of our health and well-being. I've been there too, caught in the hustle, feeling like there's never enough time for self-care.

This book is here to change that narrative. The primary goal is to empower you to achieve holistic wellness through mindful nutrition, exercise, and sustainable lifestyle changes. Think of it as your friendly guide, offering practical advice and helping you build habits that last. No more fads or quick fixes—just real solutions that fit into your busy life.

What makes this book unique is its interactive approach. It's not just a read-and-forget kind of book. It's a guided journal designed for active participation. You'll find prompts for self-reflection, goal setting, and even curated music suggestions to make your journey more enjoyable. By the end of each chapter, you'll have a personalized map of your own wellness path.

Who will benefit from this journey? Whether you're navigating the demands of a burgeoning career, managing the whirlwind of parenthood, or adjusting to a new chapter in your life, this guide is crafted with you in mind. You prioritize personal development and seek authentic, feasible strategies for self-care amidst a schedule brimming with obligations.

The themes we'll explore together are interconnected: mindful eating, holistic fitness, and sustainable weight loss. Each plays a crucial role in your journey toward comprehensive well-being. Mindful eating encourages you to appreciate your food and understand its impact on your body. Holistic fitness focuses on exercises that you enjoy and can maintain. Sustainable weight loss is about making changes that stick, without feeling deprived.

I know the struggle of sifting through conflicting health advice. It can be confusing and overwhelming, especially when time and motivation are in short supply. This book addresses these common pain points by offering clear, actionable solutions. It's about cutting through the noise and finding what truly works for you.

Let's talk about how this book is structured. We'll start with foundational concepts that set the stage for your wellness journey. Each chapter progresses to practical applications, complete with journal prompts and exercises to encourage self-discovery and habit formation. You'll learn how to integrate these practices into your daily routine effortlessly.

This guide is designed to be practical and accessible. The advice here is easy to follow and meant to be adapted to your lifestyle, regardless of your current fitness level or experience with wellness practices. Whether you're just starting or looking to deepen your current routine, you'll find something valuable here.

As you engage with this book, you'll begin to see a transformation. You'll discover that holistic health is not only attainable but also empowering. Mindful living will become second nature, and you'll feel more balanced and energized. You'll gain the confidence to take control of your health in a way that feels right for you.

So, let's embark on this journey together. You have the tools you need within these pages to create a life that supports your well-being. Take a deep breath, turn the page, and step into a world where health and happiness coexist, even amidst the busyness of life.

Chapter 1

Embracing the Mind-Body Connection

You know those days when your body feels like it's on autopilot, ticking off tasks without a second thought? You might be checking emails during breakfast, squeezing in a quick workout between meetings, and mindlessly snacking while trying to meet deadlines. We've all had days like that, feeling like we're just going through the motions without being truly present. This chapter invites you to press pause on that chaos. It's a gentle nudge to reconnect with yourself—not just physically, but mentally and emotionally too. It's about finding harmony in a world that often feels anything but balanced. Here, we'll explore how embracing the connection between your mind and body can transform your approach to fitness and wellness.

Understanding Holistic Fitness

Holistic fitness is not just another trend. It's a comprehensive approach that emphasizes the interconnectedness of your body, mind, and inner self. Imagine a fitness regime where strength, mental clarity, and emotional resilience are equally prioritized. This approach is about achieving harmony across all aspects of health, rather than focusing solely on physical appearance or performance. It's about recognizing that your mental and emotional well-being are just as important as your physical strength. By integrating body, mind, and spirit, you create a balanced lifestyle that nurtures every part of you. This balance can lead to lasting health benefits, helping you navigate life with a sense of calm and purpose.

Traditional fitness models often fall short when it comes to addressing overall well-being. They tend to overemphasize physical appearance, promoting the idea that fitness is solely about achieving a certain look. This focus can neglect the mental health components that are crucial for sustained wellness. When exercise becomes solely about aesthetics, it can lead to burnout, dissatisfaction, and a disconnect between body and mind. Holistic fitness, on the other hand, promotes a balanced approach that considers the whole person. It encourages you to move with intention, focusing on how exercise makes you feel rather than just how it makes you look.

Balance is the cornerstone of holistic fitness. It involves giving equal importance to strength, flexibility, and endurance. Each component contributes to overall health and wellness, ensuring that your body is well-rounded and capable of handling various physical demands. Strength training builds muscle and bone density, while flexibility exercises like yoga improve range of motion and prevent injuries. Endurance activities, such as running or cycling, enhance cardiovascular health and stamina. Together, these elements create a fitness routine that supports your body's needs, helping you feel strong, agile, and resilient.

Mindfulness plays a crucial role in achieving a holistic fitness regime. Mindful movement practices encourage you to be present during exercise, focusing on the sensations in your body and the rhythm of your breath. This awareness helps you connect with your body on a deeper level, enhancing the effectiveness of your workouts. Mindfulness also promotes mental clarity, which is essential for staying motivated and committed to your fitness goals. When you exercise with mindfulness, you cultivate a sense of inner peace and focus that extends beyond the gym. It becomes a practice that nourishes your mind and spirit, leaving you feeling rejuvenated and centered.

Reflection Journal

Consider your current fitness routine. Reflect on how much of it focuses solely on physical appearance versus overall well-being. Jot down any changes you'd like to make to incorporate more mindfulness and balance. How can you better integrate strength, flexibility, and endurance into your routine? What small steps can you take to ensure your workouts nourish both your body and mind? This exercise is a starting point for embracing holistic fitness, helping you create a plan that aligns with your values and lifestyle.

Reflection on My Current Fitness Routine Take a moment to reflect: How much of your current routine is focused on physical appearance? How much supports your overall well-being? Are you satisfied with the balance?

My thoughts:

Changes I'd Like to Make Think about how you can bring more mindfulness and balance into your routine. What areas feel neglected? How can you shift your focus to activities that nourish both body and mind?

I'd like to:

Building Strength, Flexibility, and Endurance Consider ways to incorporate these three pillars into your fitness plan. What activities feel enjoyable and sustainable for you?

- **Strength:**

- **Flexibility:**

- **Endurance:**

Small Steps Toward Holistic Fitness What small, actionable changes can you start today or this week? Reflect on ways to make your workouts more intentional and aligned with your values.

My next steps:

Final Thoughts How do you feel after reflecting on your fitness routine? What motivates you to make these changes? What impact do you hope this holistic approach will have on your life?

Closing thoughts:

Music Suggestion Enhance your reflection or workout experience with music that inspires mindfulness and energy. Try:

- **Instrumental Focus:** *Weightless* by Marconi Union

- **Mindful Energy:** *Aloha Ke Akua* by Nahko and Medicine for the People

- **Strength & Power:** *Eye of the Tiger* by Survivor

- **Relaxation & Stretching:** *Clair de Lune* by Debussy

The Science of Mindfulness in Exercise

Imagine you're in the middle of a workout, your mind racing with thoughts of unfinished tasks and looming deadlines. Yet, as you settle into the rhythm of your movements, something shifts. You focus on your breath, the sensation of your muscles contracting and releasing, and the gentle beat of your heart. This is mindfulness in exercise, a practice that transforms a routine workout into a meditative experience. Scientifically, mindfulness during exercise reduces cortisol levels, the notorious stress hormone that often keeps us in a state of constant tension. Lowering cortisol not only eases stress but also enhances focus and concentration, allowing you to be fully present in each movement. When your mind is clear, your workouts become more efficient, and you find yourself moving with purpose rather than obligation. This enhanced focus creates a positive loop, improving your muscle relaxation and overall performance. With each mindful breath, you become more in tune with your body's needs, fostering a sense of calm and control.

On the neurological front, mindfulness in exercise plays a fascinating role. Engaging in mindful practices can increase neuroplasticity, the brain's ability to adapt and reorganize itself. This adaptability translates into enhanced memory and learning, crucial benefits for those of us juggling countless responsibilities. Picture your brain as a muscle—it strengthens with use, becoming more adept at handling complex tasks and retaining new information. When you integrate mindfulness into your exercise routine, you're not just training your body but also sharpening your brain. Studies have shown that mindfulness-based interventions can significantly improve cognitive performance, helping you tackle daily challenges with newfound clarity and creativity. As your brain becomes more efficient, you might notice an improvement in decision-making and problem-solving, skills that are invaluable in both personal and professional settings.

Mental health, too, reaps the rewards of mindfulness in exercise. Regular practice can lead to a reduction in symptoms of anxiety and depression, offering a natural and empowering way to manage mental health. By focusing on the present moment, you create a mental space free from worry and fear. This presence allows you to connect with your emotions, understand them, and let go of those that do not serve you. Engaging in mindful workouts can become a form of moving meditation, where the act of exercising becomes a powerful tool for nurturing mental well-being.

As mindfulness practices take root, you'll likely experience an increase in self-compassion and acceptance, fostering a healthier relationship with yourself and your body.

So, how do we bring mindfulness into our exercise routines? Mindful yoga sequences are a brilliant place to start. Yoga emphasizes breath control and awareness of the body, encouraging you to move with intention. Each pose becomes an opportunity to explore your body's capabilities and limitations without judgment. Focused breathing, a core component of yoga, further enhances the connection between mind and body. Alternatively, consider incorporating breathing-focused aerobic activities, such as walking or running, where the rhythm of your breath guides each step. These activities encourage a meditative state, allowing you to immerse yourself in the flow of movement and breath. The goal is not to achieve perfection but to cultivate a practice that supports both physical fitness and mental clarity.

Mindful Movement Journal

Next time you head out for a run or walk, try this mindful exercise: as you begin, focus on the sensation of your feet touching the ground. Feel the texture beneath you and the rhythm of your steps. Gradually bring your attention to your breath, matching its pace with the movement. If your mind starts to wander, gently bring it back to the present moment. Notice the sights, sounds, and sensations around you. This simple exercise transforms a *routine activity into an opportunity for mindfulness, helping you connect with yourself and the world in a meaningful way.*

Reflection on My Current Movement Practice Take a moment to consider your usual approach to walking or running. How present are you during these activities? Do you often find your mind wandering, or are you fully engaged with the experience?

My thoughts:

Intentions for Mindful Movement Think about how you can bring more mindfulness to your next walk or run. What sensations, rhythms, or surroundings would you like to focus on?

I'd like to focus on:

Mindful Movement Exercise The next time you go for a walk or run, try the following steps:

- **Feet:** Focus on the sensation of your feet touching the ground. What does the texture beneath you feel like? *My experience:*

- **Breath:** Bring attention to your breath. Can you match its pace with your steps? *My experience:*

- **Mindfulness:** If your thoughts wander, gently guide

them back to the present. Notice the sights, sounds, and sensations around you. *My experience:*

Small Steps to Make This a Habit What can you do to integrate this practice into your routine? How can you remind yourself to stay mindful during movement?
My next steps:

Final Thoughts How did this exercise make you feel? What insights or feelings came up during your mindful movement?
Closing thoughts:

Music Suggestion Enhance your mindful movement with music that complements your pace and helps you stay present:

- **For a Calm Walk:** *River Flows in You* by Yiruma

- **For an Energizing Run:** *Adventure of a Lifetime* by Coldplay

- **For Nature Walks:** *Morning Mood* by Edvard Grieg

- **For Focus and Grounding:** *Bloom* by ODESZA

Cultivating Awareness in Movement

When was the last time you truly paid attention to how your body moved? Maybe you were rushing through a workout, barely noticing how your muscles engaged and released. Awareness in movement invites you to change that perspective. It's about consciously engaging your muscles and paying attention to your form and posture. This level of awareness can transform exercise from a monotonous task to a mindful practice. By noticing the way your body moves, you create a deeper connection with it, enhancing the effectiveness of your workouts. It's like shifting from autopilot to manual mode, where each movement becomes intentional and meaningful.

Developing this awareness requires practice, but the benefits are well worth the effort. One technique is body scanning during workouts. This involves mentally checking in with different parts of your body as you move, noticing any tension or discomfort. It's about being present in each moment, focusing on the sensation of your muscles contracting and relaxing. Visualization exercises can also enhance awareness. Picture the muscles you're working, visualize their movement and imagine the energy flowing through them. These techniques help you engage more deeply with your body, improving your form and alignment.

Increased movement awareness can prevent injuries and enhance performance. Proper alignment and posture reduce the risk of strains and sprains, allowing you to exercise safely and effectively. When you're aware of how your body moves, you can make adjustments that prevent overexertion and imbalances. This awareness also enhances proprioception, your body's ability to sense its position and movement in space. Improved proprioception means greater balance and coordination, helping you move with confidence and precision.

Consider incorporating exercises that focus on building awareness into your routine. Tai Chi, for example, is a practice that emphasizes slow, deliberate movements, promoting balance and control. Each movement flows into the next, encouraging you to focus on the present moment and the sensations in your body. Pilates is another excellent choice, as it emphasizes core awareness and alignment. The controlled movements require you to engage your muscles intentionally, fostering a deep connection between your mind and body.

Visualization Journal

Try this visualization exercise during your next workout. As you perform each movement, close your eyes for a moment and imagine the muscles you're engaging. Visualize them contracting and releasing, picture the energy flowing through them, and focus on the sensations in your body. This technique helps you tune into your body's needs, enhancing your awareness and improving your performance.

Reflection on My Mind-Body Connection Think about how connected you feel to your body during workouts. Do you often focus on the movements and sensations, or are you distracted by other thoughts?

My thoughts:

Intentions for Visualization Consider how incorporating visualization can improve your awareness and performance. What aspects of your workout do you want to focus on more deeply?

I'd like to focus on:

Visualization Exercise During your next workout, follow these steps to engage in visualization:

- **Close Your Eyes Momentarily:** As you perform each movement, take a moment to close your eyes (if it's safe to do so). *What I noticed:*

- **Visualize the Muscles Engaging:** Imagine the specific muscles you're using, contracting and releasing with each motion. *What I felt:*

- **Picture Energy Flowing:** Envision energy coursing through your body, fueling your movements and enhancing your strength. *My experience:*

- **Focus on Sensations:** Pay attention to the feelings in your body—the stretch, tension, and release. *My sensations:*

Small Steps to Make This a Habit How can you regularly incorporate visualization into your workouts? What reminders or tools could help you stay mindful?
My next steps:

Final Thoughts Reflect on how this visualization exercise impacted your workout. Did it change the way you experienced your movements? How did it affect your focus or performance?
Closing thoughts:

Music Suggestion Pair your visualization exercise with music that enhances focus and body awareness:

- **For Deep Focus:** *Weightless* by Marconi Union

- **For Slow, Controlled Movements:** *Nuvole Bianche* by

Ludovico Einaudi

- **For Energized Visualization:** *On Top of the World* by Imagine Dragons

- **For Centered Strength:** *Rise* by Hans Zimmer

Cultivating awareness in movement is about more than just exercise. It's a practice that extends into everyday life, helping you move through the world with intention and grace. Whether you're walking to work, lifting groceries, or playing with your kids, this awareness invites you to be present in each moment. It encourages you to appreciate the capabilities of your body and the joy of movement, creating a sense of gratitude and connection.

Breathing Techniques for Mental Clarity

Ever notice how a few deep breaths can change your entire perspective on a stressful situation? There's more to it than just a temporary sense of calm. The way we breathe affects our mental clarity and focus. When you take a deep breath, you're not just filling your lungs with air. You're oxygenating your brain, which is crucial for clear thinking and decision-making. This simple act also calms the nervous system by activating the parasympathetic nervous system, which is responsible for resting and digesting. It's like hitting the reset button for your mind, helping to clear away the fog that stress and anxiety often bring.

Let's explore some specific breathing exercises that can help enhance this mental clarity. Diaphragmatic breathing, or deep belly breathing, is a powerful technique. To try it, place one hand on your chest and the other on your belly. As you inhale deeply through your nose, your belly should rise more than your chest. This technique encourages full oxygen exchange, slows the heartbeat, and can lower or stabilize blood pressure. Another effective method is the 4-7-8 breathing technique. Start by breathing in quietly through your nose for four seconds, hold the breath for seven seconds, and then exhale completely through your mouth for eight seconds. This exercise is known to calm the mind, reduce anxiety, and help you fall asleep faster.

Breathing correctly can significantly reduce stress. When you're stressed, your body tends to take shallow, rapid breaths. This kind of breathing signals the fight-or-flight response, keeping the body in a state of alertness. By practicing proper breathing techniques, you can reverse this response, reducing physical tension and lowering your heart rate. It's amazing how something as simple as altering your breath can bring about such profound changes. Try these techniques next time you feel overwhelmed, and notice the difference in how your body responds to stress.

Breath control is not just about mental clarity; it also plays a crucial role in physical performance. Athletes and fitness enthusiasts know the importance of breathing techniques for improving endurance and efficiency. When you manage your breath, you optimize oxygen delivery to your muscles, which increases endurance and performance. Think of it like ensuring a steady flow of fuel to an engine. Efficient oxygen use means you can sustain activity for longer periods without exhaustion. Whether you're running a marathon or simply going for a brisk walk, mastering these techniques can give you that extra boost.

Breathing Journal

Try incorporating a simple breathing exercise into your daily routine. Set aside a few minutes each morning to practice diaphragmatic breathing. As you wake up, sit comfortably and close your eyes. Focus on taking deep, slow breaths, letting your mind clear as you inhale and exhale. This small practice can set a positive tone for the rest of your day, enhancing your focus and reducing stress. Remember, your breath is a powerful tool for achieving mental clarity and balance, so make it a part of your wellness toolkit.

Reflection on My Current Breathing Habits How often do you pay attention to your breath throughout the day? Do you notice any connection between your breathing and your stress or focus levels?

Intentions for Mindful Breathing What benefits do you hope to gain from practicing diaphragmatic breathing? How can this exercise support your overall well-being?

Breathing Exercise Incorporate this practice into your routine:
- **Start the Day with Breath:** Sit comfortably and close your eyes.
- **Focus on Your Breathing:** Take deep, slow breaths, feeling your diaphragm expand as you inhale and contract as you exhale.
- **Clear Your Mind:** Let go of any thoughts and simply be present with each breath.

Small Steps to Build a Habit How can you make this breathing exercise a consistent part of your day? What reminders or adjustments to your schedule might help?

Final Thoughts How did you feel after practicing this exercise? Did it impact your focus, mood, or stress levels? How might regular practice enhance your day-to-day life?

Music Suggestion Pair your breathing exercise with calming music to deepen the relaxation:

- **For Calm and Centering:** *Quiet Resource* by Liquid Mind

- **For Gentle Mornings:** *Prelude in E Minor* by Chopin

- **For Stress Reduction:** *Breathe* by Moby

Body Scanning for Stress Reduction

Picture yourself lying comfortably on your back, eyes gently closed, as you begin to tune into the rhythm of your breath. This simple yet profound practice is known as body scanning, a mindfulness meditation technique that encourages you to scan your body for any signs of pain, tension, or anything that feels out of the ordinary. Body scanning invites you to explore the connection between physical sensations and your mental state, fostering a sense of awareness that often gets lost in the hustle of daily life. By gradually shifting your attention from one part of your body to another, you cultivate a deeper understanding of how stress manifests physically. This awareness is the first step towards releasing chronic tension and promoting relaxation.

To begin, find a quiet space where you won't be disturbed. Lie down on a comfortable surface, such as a yoga mat or your bed, and close your eyes. Start by taking a few deep breaths, allowing your body to settle into relaxation. Slowly direct your attention to your toes, noticing any sensations without judgment. Perhaps you feel warmth, tingling, or tension. With each exhale, imagine any tension melting away. Gradually move your focus upward, from your feet to your ankles, calves, knees, and so on, until you reach the top of your head. As you scan each area, acknowledge any sensations you encounter, sending a breath of relaxation to those areas. The goal isn't to change anything but to simply notice and accept what is present.

Regular practice of body scanning can lead to significant stress reduction over time. By consistently checking in with your body, you train yourself to recognize and release tension before it becomes chronic. This practice enhances your relaxation response, a state where your body can restore itself and heal. The more you engage in body scanning, the more adept you become at recognizing early signs of stress, allowing you to take proactive steps to manage it. Imagine being able to catch yourself before stress spirals out of control, simply by tuning into the language of your body. This kind of self-awareness is empowering, giving you the tools to navigate stress with grace and confidence.

Body scanning is versatile and can be incorporated into various contexts throughout your day. Consider using it during the cool-down phase of your workout, when your body is already in a relaxed state and receptive to mindfulness. As you transition from movement to stillness, take a few minutes to scan your body, acknowledging the work it has done and releasing any residual tension. Alternatively, make body scanning a part of your daily mindfulness practice. Set aside a few moments each morning or evening to reconnect with your body, allowing this practice to become a soothing ritual that anchors your day. Whether you're winding down after a long day or preparing for the challenges ahead, body scanning offers a moment of peace and introspection.

Incorporating body scanning into your routine doesn't require any special equipment or expertise. It's a practice that meets you where you are, inviting you to pause and listen to the wisdom of your body. As you cultivate this awareness, you'll find that the boundaries between your physical sensations and mental states blur, revealing the intricate connection between body and mind. This practice not only reduces stress but also deepens your relationship with yourself, fostering a sense of compassion and understanding. As you continue to explore body scanning, you'll discover its potential to transform your experience of stress, guiding you towards a more mindful and balanced life.

Integrating Mindfulness into Daily Routines

Imagine waking up and feeling like you're fully present with each moment. The hum of the morning bustle doesn't overwhelm you but instead feels like a gentle reminder that you're alive. Mindfulness can bring this sense of presence and awareness into our daily routines. It's about creating habits that support mental and emotional well-being, allowing us to navigate life's challenges with grace. Integrating mindfulness into everyday life isn't about making drastic changes. It's about embedding small, consistent practices that sustain us, providing continuous support for our mental and emotional health. When mindfulness becomes a part of our daily routine, it lays the foundation for sustainable habits that foster holistic wellness.

Incorporating mindfulness doesn't have to be complicated. It can begin with mindful eating practices during meals. This means truly tasting and savoring each bite, paying attention to flavors and textures without distraction. By slowing down and engaging with your food, you create a moment of connection with yourself, turning an everyday activity into a mindful experience. Another simple yet profound practice is gratitude. Taking a moment each day to acknowledge what you're grateful for can shift your perspective and foster a positive mindset. It could be something as small as the warmth of your morning coffee or the smile of a loved one. These acts of mindfulness anchor us in the present, reminding us of the abundance in our lives.

The benefits of consistent mindfulness are profound. Regular practice can improve emotional regulation, helping us respond to situations with calm and clarity rather than reacting impulsively. It enhances overall satisfaction and well-being, allowing us to appreciate life's small joys and navigate challenges with resilience. As mindfulness becomes a regular practice, it cultivates a sense of peace and contentment that permeates every aspect of our lives. We begin to notice the beauty in the ordinary and find happiness in simplicity, creating a ripple effect that positively influences our relationships and interactions.

To enhance your mindfulness journey, explore the array of mindfulness tools and resources available. Apps designed for beginners feature guided meditations and timely reminders, serving as an invaluable aid to maintain consistency in your practice. These digital companions provide a solid foundation, guiding you gently into the realm of mindfulness. Additionally, recordings of guided meditations present another avenue to deepen your practice, offering expert-led instructions that you can follow at your own pace. Regardless of how much time you can dedicate—be it a brief five-minute pause or an extended hour-long session—these resources seamlessly integrate into your daily routine, ensuring mindfulness is both accessible and practical for your lifestyle.

As you integrate mindfulness into your routine, you'll find that it becomes a natural part of your day, like brushing your teeth or having your morning coffee. It's about creating a rhythm that aligns with your lifestyle, making mindfulness a seamless part of who you are. Over time, mindfulness transforms from a practice into a way of being, enriching your life with presence and purpose. You'll notice a shift in how you perceive and interact with the world, feeling more grounded and connected.

Incorporating mindfulness into daily life doesn't require perfection. It's a journey of exploration, where each day offers an opportunity to learn and grow. Some days you may feel deeply connected, while others may be more challenging. Embrace each experience with curiosity and compassion, knowing that mindfulness is a practice that evolves with you. As you continue to cultivate mindfulness, you'll find that it enhances your overall well-being, providing a steady anchor amidst the ebb and flow of life. Embrace mindfulness as a companion on your path, guiding you towards a life of balance and fulfillment.

Chapter 2

Mindful Nutrition Essentials

Sitting at your desk, the laptop's glow reflects in the room, accompanied by the relentless ticking of the clock. Hours have slipped away, and you find yourself reaching for another snack on autopilot. This scenario is all too familiar for many of us—eating without awareness, hardly noticing as the food quickly vanishes. This habit of mindless eating, driven by convenience rather than genuine enjoyment, is a pattern many fall into. However, it's possible to rewrite this script. Mindful eating presents a compelling alternative, centering on the full sensory experience of our meals rather than solely their calorie content or nutritional value. This method encourages a full engagement with what we eat, taking the time to relish each bite and truly appreciate the taste and texture of our food. It transforms eating from a routine task into an act of mindfulness, creating a moment to connect deeply with our food and ourselves, and nurturing a more positive relationship with both.

Mindful eating is a practice that emphasizes awareness, encouraging you to slow down and truly notice what you're eating. Unlike traditional eating patterns, which often prioritize speed and efficiency, mindful eating asks you to pause and engage your senses. It's about tuning into the taste, smell, and even sound of your food. This practice helps reduce mindless eating habits, which can be unhealthy and often lead to overeating. When meals become an automatic, hurried act, you lose the ability to recognize when you're truly satisfied, leading to unnecessary consumption. Mindful eating, on the other hand, cultivates a sense of presence, allowing you to enjoy your food without distraction and recognize when you've had enough.

The benefits of mindful eating extend beyond mere enjoyment. One significant advantage is improved digestion. When you eat slowly, your body has more time to signal fullness, and your digestive system can process food more effectively. This slower pace can reduce discomfort and bloating, common issues when meals are rushed. Mindful eating also leads to greater satisfaction with smaller portions. By paying attention to the experience of eating, you become more attuned to your body's signals, realizing you need less to feel content. This can naturally lead to healthier portion control and a more balanced diet.

So how do you start practicing mindful eating? It begins with setting a calm, distraction-free environment. Create a space where you can focus solely on your meal, free from the usual interruptions of screens and noise. Before you take your first bite, ask yourself a few questions: Why are you eating right now? Are you truly hungry, or are you eating out of habit or emotion? Consider the nutritional value of what you're about to consume. These questions help ground you in the present moment and align your eating with your body's actual needs.

Mindful eating can be seamlessly integrated into various aspects of your daily life. Take snacking during work breaks, for example. Instead of mindlessly munching while checking emails, dedicate a few minutes to really taste your snack. Notice the texture, the flavors, and how it makes you feel. This practice transforms a quick snack into a nourishing pause, recharging your body and mind. Dining out is another opportunity to practice mindfulness. When you're at a restaurant, take a moment before eating to admire the presentation of your dish. Engage with each bite, savoring the chef's craft, and enjoy the company of those around you without rushing through the meal.

Reflection Journal

Consider your last meal. Reflect on how you approached it—were you mindful or distracted? What was the environment like? Take a moment to jot down your thoughts and any changes you'd like to implement. How can you make your next meal a more mindful experience? What steps will you take to ensure you're present, engaged, and truly enjoying your food? This reflection is the first step in cultivating a mindful eating practice that supports both your physical health and emotional well-being.

Reflection on My Last Meal Think about your most recent meal. Were you mindful or distracted? What was the environment like? How did you feel during and after the meal?

Changes I'd Like to Make Consider how you can approach your next meal more mindfully. What adjustments to your environment, mindset, or habits would help you stay present and engaged?

Creating a Mindful Eating Practice As you plan your next meal, think about the following:

- **Preparation:** How can you create a calm and inviting space for your meal?

- **Engagement:** What can you focus on while eating (e.g., flavors, textures, gratitude)?

- **Presence:** What distractions can you minimize to stay fully in the moment?

Small Steps to Build the Habit What small, actionable steps can you take to incorporate mindful eating into your daily routine?

Final Thoughts How does reflecting on your eating habits make you feel? What benefits do you hope to gain by cultivating a mindful eating practice?

Music Suggestion Enhance your mindful eating experience with soothing background music:

- **For Calm and Relaxation:** *Canon in D* by Pachelbel
- **For a Peaceful Atmosphere:** *Pure Shores* by All Saints
- **For Gratitude and Reflection:** *Thank You* by Alanis Morissette

Building a Balanced Plate with Intention

Creating a balanced plate isn't just about filling your plate with random foods or sticking strictly to calorie counts. It's about ensuring that each meal is a harmonious blend of nutrients that cater to your body's needs. Imagine your plate as a canvas, and you're the artist. On one side, you have proteins—lean meats, fish, beans, or tofu—that work to build and repair tissues. A quarter of your plate should hold these powerhouses. Then there are the carbohydrates, which are your main energy source. Think whole grains like brown rice, quinoa, or barley. These should fill another quarter. Healthy fats, though small in portion, play a crucial role in absorbing vitamins. These can come from olive oil, avocados, or nuts. Finally, fill half your plate with a vibrant array of fruits and vegetables. They not only add color and texture but provide essential vitamins, minerals, and fiber that keep your body running smoothly. By focusing on variety, you ensure that your meals are not only nutritious but also appealing and satisfying.

Meal planning is more than just a chore—it's a powerful tool to help you make healthier choices and achieve your nutritional goals. By taking the time to plan meals ahead, you can avoid the temptation of last-minute, unhealthy food decisions that often arise from a busy lifestyle. When you're exhausted and the fridge is empty, having a planned meal ready to cook offers a quick, nutritious alternative to takeout. Planning meals also ensures your diet stays varied and balanced, helping you incorporate seasonal produce, which is fresher and often more affordable. With intentional meal planning, you can effortlessly meet your nutritional needs and enjoy diverse, exciting meals without the stress of figuring out what to eat each day.

When building balanced meals, consider using the plate method as a practical guide for portion control. This method offers a visual representation of how different food groups should be proportioned on your plate. Imagine dividing your plate into sections: half for fruits and vegetables, a quarter for proteins, and a quarter for whole grains. This simple strategy helps you maintain balance without overthinking. Another tip is to incorporate seasonal produce, which ensures a variety of nutrients and flavors in your diet. Seasonal fruits and vegetables are often fresher and more nutrient-dense, making them a healthy and flavorful addition to meals. They also tend to be more affordable and environmentally friendly, as they require less transportation and storage.

Here are a couple of meal ideas to inspire your balanced plate creations. Start with grilled chicken, seasoned to perfection, paired with fluffy quinoa. Add a hearty serving of roasted vegetables like bell peppers, zucchini, and carrots, lightly tossed in olive oil and herbs for a flavorful, nutrient-rich meal.

For a plant-based option, try a lentil salad. Mix nutrient-dense lentils with fresh greens, cherry tomatoes, cucumber slices, and a touch of red onion. Top it off with a citrus vinaigrette for a refreshing and satisfying dish packed with protein, fiber, and vibrant flavors.

Reflection Journal

Take a moment to reflect on your current meal patterns. Are there areas where you could introduce more variety or balance? Consider the foods you typically consume and envision ways to incorporate more colors and textures. Write down three changes you could make this week to create a more balanced plate. Perhaps it's trying a new vegetable, experimenting with a different grain, or simply adjusting portion sizes. Small shifts can make a big difference in your nutritional intake and overall health.

Reflection on My Current Meal Patterns Take a moment to think about the foods you typically consume. Are there areas where you notice a lack of variety or balance? How do you feel about the choices you've been making?

Introducing Variety and Balance How can you incorporate more colors, textures, and nutrients into your meals? What small shifts could enhance the overall quality of your diet?

Three Changes for This Week Write down three specific changes you'd like to make to create a more balanced plate:

Small Steps Toward Better Nutrition What small, actionable steps can you take today to start implementing these changes?

Final Thoughts How do you feel about making these adjustments? What impact do you hope these changes will have on your health and well-being?

Music Suggestion Enhance your reflection with calming and uplifting music:
- **For Peaceful Focus:** *Morning Light* by Norah Jones
- **For Creative Inspiration:** *Clair de Lune* by Debussy
- **For Motivation and Positivity:** *Here Comes the Sun* by The Beatles

Recognizing Hunger and Fullness Cues

Have you ever found yourself opening the fridge, not because you're hungry but because you're bored or stressed? Differentiating between physical and emotional hunger is key to maintaining a healthy relationship with food. Physical hunger comes on gradually, and it can be satisfied with almost any food. It's your body's way of signaling that it needs fuel. Emotional hunger, on the other hand, is sudden and often tied to specific cravings. It might lead you to reach for comfort foods that give a temporary sense of relief but leave you feeling unsatisfied. Recognizing these cues is crucial, as it allows you to respond to your body's true needs rather than its emotional desires.

Tuning into your hunger and fullness cues can transform your eating habits. When you learn to recognize satiety, you're less likely to overeat, which helps maintain a healthy weight and reduces the risk of digestive discomfort. This awareness also supports regular meal timing, preventing the cycle of extreme hunger followed by overeating. By responding to your body's natural signals, you create a balanced eating pattern that keeps your energy levels steady throughout the day. It's like listening to your internal clock, which knows when it's time to fuel up and when it's time to stop. This harmony with your body's rhythms fosters both physical and emotional well-being.

To enhance your awareness of these cues, consider keeping a hunger and fullness journal. Before and after each meal, jot down your hunger level on a scale from one to ten, with one being ravenous and ten being uncomfortably full. This practice helps you become more attuned to your body's signals, making it easier to distinguish between true hunger and other triggers. Another technique is to practice mindful breathing before meals. Take a moment to breathe deeply, tuning into your body and assessing your hunger level. This pause creates a space for reflection, allowing you to make conscious choices about what and how much to eat. These practices foster a deeper connection with your body, empowering you to eat with intention and awareness.

Real-life challenges can often blur these signals. Imagine a typical workday filled with back-to-back meetings and looming deadlines. It's easy to fall into the trap of distracted eating, where meals become an afterthought rather than a mindful act. In such scenarios, setting designated meal times can help. Even if it's just ten minutes, make sure to step away from your desk and focus solely on your meal. Emotional triggers, such as stress or anxiety, can also mask true hunger. On a stressful day, you might find yourself reaching for food as a distraction or comfort. Recognizing these patterns is the first step to addressing them. Instead of turning to food, explore alternative coping mechanisms like a quick walk or a few minutes of meditation. These practices can provide the emotional relief you're seeking without relying on food.

Reflection Journal

Take a moment to reflect on your recent meals. Consider how often you eat out of hunger versus emotion. Are there particular triggers that lead to emotional eating? Write down your observations and any patterns you notice. Identifying these triggers is the first step in addressing them, helping you cultivate a more mindful approach to eating.

Reflection on My Recent Meals Think about your recent meals. How often do you eat when you're genuinely hungry, and how often is it driven by emotions? Are there specific emotions or situations that trigger you to eat?

Identifying Emotional Eating Triggers Reflect on the moments that may have led to emotional eating. What emotions or circumstances prompt you to eat, even when you're not physically hungry?

Recognizing Patterns Are there recurring situations or feelings that influence your eating habits? How do these patterns affect your relationship with food and your overall well-being?

Small Steps Toward Mindful Eating What small actions can you take to create more awareness around emotional eating? How can you respond to emotional triggers without turning to food?

Final Thoughts How does reflecting on your emotional eating patterns make you feel? What insights have you gained, and how do you plan to approach your meals differently moving forward?

Music Suggestion Pair this exercise with calming music to help center your thoughts:

- **For Reflection and Calm:** *Weightless* by Marconi Union

- **For Clarity and Focus:** *River Flows in You* by Yiruma

- **For Grounding:** *The Sound of Silence* by Simon & Garfunkel

Savoring Food: Techniques for Slowing Down

A meal can be a moment of calm amidst the chaos of the day, offering a chance to pause and appreciate the simple pleasure of nourishment. The table is set, the aroma of freshly cooked food fills the air, and that first bite invites you to savor the flavors and textures. Savoring food is about more than just eating; it's about slowing down to fully engage with each mouthful, allowing you to enjoy the experience and enhance your connection to the food.

Slowing down also supports better digestion. Taking time to chew thoroughly helps break down food more effectively, promoting nutrient absorption and reducing the risk of bloating or discomfort. By eating mindfully, you give your body the chance to process food more efficiently, while turning a routine meal into a moment of mindfulness and enjoyment.

One effective way to slow down your eating is to put utensils down between bites. This simple action forces you to pause, giving your body time to register fullness and appreciate the meal. It might feel awkward at first, but it's a powerful tool for mindful eating. Engaging in conversation during meals is another technique. It's a natural way to pace yourself, as talking and listening prevent you from rushing through your food. By focusing on the company as well as the meal, you create a shared experience that enriches both the social and culinary aspects of dining. These methods transform eating into a leisurely activity rather than a rushed necessity, allowing you to enjoy your food and the moment fully.

The impact of savoring food goes beyond immediate satisfaction. Taking the time to enjoy your meals can significantly improve digestion. When you chew your food thoroughly, you help your digestive system do its job more effectively, breaking down nutrients and absorbing them properly. This process reduces the risk of digestive issues like bloating and discomfort, which often accompany hurried meals. Additionally, savoring food enhances your sense of fullness, allowing you to feel satisfied with less. This awareness of fullness can help prevent overeating, supporting a balanced diet and healthy weight management. By slowing down, you give your body the opportunity to communicate its needs, leading to a healthier, more enjoyable eating experience.

To practice savoring food, try engaging in mindful tasting sessions with small portions. Start with a small serving of your favorite dish, and focus on the flavors and textures as you eat. Notice the subtle nuances, the way the flavors develop, and how each bite feels. This exercise trains your senses to appreciate food more fully, enhancing your enjoyment of each meal. Another practice is mindful tea or coffee drinking rituals. Instead of gulping down your morning cup on the go, set aside a few moments to savor it. Pay attention to the aroma, the warmth of the mug in your hands, and the rich flavors as you sip. These rituals encourage you to slow down and appreciate the simple pleasures of life, turning routine tasks into moments of mindfulness.

Mindful Tasting Journal

Next time you prepare a meal, set aside a few minutes for a mindful tasting session. Serve yourself a small portion and focus on each bite. Notice the flavors, textures, and aromas. How does the food change as you chew? Take your time, putting your fork down between bites. Reflect on the experience and how it differs from eating on autopilot. By incorporating these exercises into your routine, you'll cultivate a deeper appreciation for food and a heightened sense of satisfaction from meals.

Savoring your food is an art that enriches your relationship with eating, transforming it from a necessity into a celebration of flavors and nourishment.

Reflection on My Eating Experience Next time you prepare a meal, take a moment to reflect on how you typically eat. Do you eat quickly, distracted, or mindlessly? How does that affect your overall satisfaction with the meal?

Mindful Tasting Exercise As you prepare your next meal, plan to engage in a mindful tasting session:

- **Focus on the First Bite:** Pay attention to the flavors, textures, and aromas of your food.

- **Savor Each Bite:** Take your time and notice how the food changes as you chew.

- **Pause Between Bites:** Put your fork down and breathe before taking the next bite.

Observations During Mindful Eating What did you notice about your food when you ate mindfully? Did you feel more connected to the meal? How did the experience differ from your usual eating habits?

Impact on Satisfaction and Awareness How did slowing down and being mindful of your food affect your sense of satisfaction? What new appreciation or awareness did you gain from the experience?

Small Steps to Cultivate Mindful Eating What small adjustments can you make to incorporate mindful tasting into your routine? How can you create a more intentional eating environment moving forward?

Final Thoughts How does it feel to practice mindful tasting? What benefits do you hope to experience by making it a regular habit?

Music Suggestion Pair this mindful eating experience with soothing music for relaxation and focus:
- **For Tranquil Focus:** *Sunset Lover* by Petit Biscuit
- **For Calm and Presence:** *Weightless* by Marconi Union
- **For Light and Uplifting Energy:** *Better Together* by Jack Johnson

Emotional Eating: Identifying and Overcoming Triggers

After a long day, the house is quiet, and you find yourself reaching for a bag of chips. While you're not truly hungry, the simple act of eating offers a sense of comfort, filling a need that goes beyond physical nourishment. This is the realm of emotional eating, where food becomes a response to feelings rather than hunger. Emotional eating often stems from stress, boredom, or loneliness. These emotions are powerful triggers, pushing you toward the pantry in search of solace. It's not about needing fuel; it's about filling a void or distracting from discomfort. Stress, in particular, is a common culprit. The demands of work, family, and life in general can build up, leading you to seek quick relief in the form of food. Boredom, too, can send you to the kitchen, looking for something to do or a taste to break the monotony. And when loneliness creeps in, food can feel like a friend, offering a momentary sense of connection. But this reliance on food for emotional comfort can have negative consequences, creating a cycle that's hard to break.

Emotional eating can lead to weight gain and nutritional imbalance, as the foods we reach for in these moments are often high in sugar, fat, or salt—not the most nutritious options available. This pattern can quickly spiral into a cycle of guilt and frustration. You eat to soothe emotions, then feel guilty about the choices you've made, which in turn leads to more emotional eating. It's a loop that's difficult to escape. The key to breaking free is to recognize and address the underlying emotional triggers. One strategy is to develop alternative coping mechanisms. Instead of turning to food, find other activities that offer comfort or distraction. This could be as simple as taking a walk, calling a friend, or engaging in a hobby. These activities provide a healthy outlet for emotions, helping you manage stress and boredom without relying on food. Seeking support from friends or professionals can also be invaluable. Sharing your challenges with someone who understands can offer relief and reinforce your efforts to change.

Consider real-world scenarios where emotional eating often occurs and how you might address them. Late-night snacking is a common habit, often driven by a need to unwind after a long day. To break this pattern, try creating a bedtime routine that doesn't involve food. Perhaps a warm bath or reading a book can provide the relaxation you seek. Establishing a stress-reduction plan that doesn't rely on food is crucial. This might include regular exercise, practicing mindfulness, or setting aside time each day for self-care. These practices help manage stress at its source, reducing the need to eat for emotional reasons. By identifying and addressing the triggers of emotional eating, you can build healthier habits that support both your physical and emotional well-being.

Sustainable Meal Planning and Prep

In a world that prioritizes convenience, sustainable meal planning stands out as an act of mindfulness and responsibility. It's about more than just choosing what to eat—it's about making thoughtful decisions that benefit both your health and the planet. One of the immediate benefits is the reduction of food waste and the cost savings that come with buying only what you need. This approach helps prevent spoiled produce from being thrown out, saving money and minimizing environmental impact. By focusing on seasonal, locally sourced ingredients, you not only enjoy fresher meals but also support local farmers and reduce the carbon footprint associated with transporting food long distances.

Meal prep is the practical side of sustainable planning, turning intentions into actions. Batch cooking is an excellent strategy here. By preparing large quantities of a dish and freezing portions, you ensure that you always have a healthy meal ready to go. This reduces the temptation to opt for less nutritious, quick-fix meals when time is short. Freezing meals also preserves nutrients, ensuring that you're getting the most out of your food. Another technique is utilizing leftovers creatively. Instead of letting those bits go to waste, think of them as ingredients for tomorrow's meal. Leftover roasted vegetables can become the base for a hearty soup, or extra rice can be transformed into a stir-fry. This approach not only saves food but also encourages culinary creativity, making meals more exciting and diverse.

The impact of sustainable practices on health and the environment is profound. A focus on varied diets, rich in seasonal and local produce, improves nutritional intake. You're more likely to consume a wider range of nutrients when your meals are diverse and colorful. This variety supports overall health, providing essential vitamins and minerals that your body needs to thrive. On an environmental level, these practices contribute to a lower footprint. Less waste means fewer resources are used, from the energy required to produce and transport food to the space needed to dispose of it. Every small change you make contributes to a healthier planet, creating a ripple effect that extends beyond your kitchen.

Practical tools and resources can make sustainable meal planning more accessible. Meal planning apps are a great starting point. Many offer templates that help you organize meals based on what's in your pantry, reducing unnecessary purchases. These apps often include shopping lists and recipes, streamlining the entire process. Guides to seasonal produce availability are also invaluable. They inform you about what's in season in your area, making it easier to plan meals around fresh, local ingredients. These guides not only enhance the quality of your meals but also support sustainable eating practices, aligning your diet with the natural rhythm of the seasons.

As you incorporate these sustainable practices into your routine, you'll find that they naturally lead to a more mindful and rewarding approach to food. The act of planning, prepping, and enjoying meals becomes a holistic experience, one that nourishes both body and soul. It's about creating a lifestyle that aligns with your values, one that supports your health while caring for the world around you. Sustainable eating isn't a sacrifice; it's a celebration of the abundance that nature offers, an opportunity to connect with your food in a meaningful way. As you close this chapter, reflect on the changes you can make today. Consider the impact of each meal, not just on your health, but on the planet. And as we transition to the next chapter, remember that every small step counts towards a healthier, more sustainable future.

Chapter 3

Personalized Fitness for Every Lifestyle

Imagine lacing up your sneakers, ready to begin a fitness journey that's specifically designed for your unique lifestyle. Unlike generic fitness plans, a personalized approach takes into account your individual needs, goals, and daily routines. We all have different lives—some balancing work calls with school drop-offs, others finding time for exercise during lunch breaks. This chapter will guide you in creating a fitness plan that's tailored just for you. Fitness isn't a one-size-fits-all endeavor; your journey should reflect your goals and limitations, meeting you exactly where you are.

Creating a custom fitness plan starts with a thorough self-assessment. This isn't just about your current fitness level; it's about understanding your aspirations and any hurdles you might face. Begin by reflecting on your fitness goals. Are you looking to shed a few pounds, boost your cardiovascular health, or maybe just feel more energized throughout the day? Next, assess your current fitness level. There are numerous online tools available that can help, from simple fitness tests you can do at home to more comprehensive assessments offered by local gyms or health clubs. Once you have a clear picture of your starting point and your destination, you can start setting realistic, achievable goals. Consider using a goal-setting worksheet—these are great for breaking down big ambitions into manageable steps and tracking your progress along the way.

Now that you've got your goals and current fitness level sorted, it's time to dive into the tools available to help you craft your personalized plan. The digital age offers a plethora of resources to aid in your journey. Online fitness planners are a fantastic starting point, providing structured templates that you can customize to fit your schedule. Many of these platforms allow you to input your goals and preferences, generating a plan that feels personal and achievable. Mobile apps are another invaluable resource, offering flexibility and convenience. Apps like MyFitnessPal or FitOn allow you to choose your workouts based on time, equipment, and intensity, making it easy to adapt your fitness routine as your needs evolve. These tools empower you to take control of your fitness journey, ensuring your plan grows and transforms alongside you.

To bring all these elements together, let's look at some examples of personalized fitness plans. Imagine you're a beginner focused on weight loss. Your plan might start with three days of low-impact cardio—think brisk walking or cycling—combined with two days of strength training using bodyweight exercises. Each session could be 30 minutes, fitting seamlessly into a busy schedule, with flexibility for days when life gets in the way. For someone looking to improve cardiovascular health, the plan might shift towards more aerobic exercises. Perhaps four days of moderate-intensity cardio, like swimming or jogging, paired with a weekly yoga session to enhance flexibility and reduce stress. These examples illustrate how a personalized approach can cater to diverse goals and lifestyles, transforming fitness from a chore into an integrated part of your life.

Interactive Journal: Create Your Fitness Plan

Take a moment to draft your personalized fitness plan. Begin by listing your primary fitness goals, considering both short-term and long-term ambitions. Next, assess your current fitness level using an online tool or a simple home test. With this information in hand, choose one or two online resources or apps that resonate with you. Finally, draft a weekly schedule that incorporates various exercises aligned with your goals. Remember, the key is flexibility—your plan should adapt to your life, not the other way around. This exercise is the first step in crafting a fitness journey that's uniquely yours, empowering you to take charge of your health and well-being.

Primary Fitness Goals Take a moment to reflect on your fitness journey. What are your primary fitness goals? Consider both short-term goals (e.g., improving endurance, losing weight) and long-term goals (e.g., building strength, maintaining health).

Assessing My Current Fitness Level Use an online tool or a simple home test to assess your current fitness level (e.g., endurance, strength, flexibility). Based on your findings, how would you rate your fitness today?

Online Resources or Apps What resources or apps resonate with you? How can they support your goals and provide guidance along the way?

Drafting My Weekly Fitness Schedule Create a weekly fitness plan that includes a balance of exercises. Consider strength, flexibility, endurance, and recovery. How many days a week will you work out, and what exercises will you focus on each day?

- **Monday:**

- **Tuesday:**

- **Wednesday:**

- **Thursday:**

- **Friday:**

- **Saturday:**

- **Sunday (Rest/Recovery):**

Flexibility and Adaptability How will you adjust your plan if life gets busy? What strategies will help you stay flexible while remaining consistent with your fitness journey?

Final Thoughts How do you feel about your personalized fitness plan? What steps will you take to implement it and make progress toward your goals?

Music Suggestion Pair your fitness journey with energizing music:

- **For Motivation:** *Stronger* by Kanye West

- **For Focus and Flow:** *Eye of the Tiger* by Survivor

- **For Recovery and Relaxation:** *Weightless* by Marconi Union

Time-Efficient Workouts for Busy Schedules

You've got a million things on your to-do list, and finding time for a workout can feel like just another impossible task. That's where time-efficient workouts come in, designed for those of us who need to squeeze fitness into the cracks of our day. These workouts are not just quick; they're effective, maximizing effort in a short span. High-intensity interval training (HIIT) is a powerhouse in this realm, alternating between bursts of intense activity and brief rest periods. This method not only boosts your metabolism but also keeps your heart rate up, burning calories long after you've finished. Circuit training is another gem, combining strength and cardio with minimal rest. It keeps your body guessing and your muscles engaged, offering a full-body workout in record time.

Here's an itemized approach to both routines for a more structured, guided experience:

20-Minute Full-Body HIIT Session

1. **Warm-up (3 minutes)**
    - High knees (1 minute)
    - Jumping jacks (1 minute)
    - Arm circles (1 minute)

2. **Main Circuit (12 minutes)**
    - Burpees (30 seconds)
    - Rest (30 seconds)
    - Squats (30 seconds)
    - Rest (30 seconds)
    - Push-ups (30 seconds)
    - Rest (30 seconds)
    - Mountain climbers (30 seconds)
    - Rest (30 seconds)
    - Repeat the circuit 2-3 times

3. **Cool-down (5 minutes)**

    - Forward fold stretch (1 minute)
    - Child's pose (1 minute)
    - Cat-cow stretch (1 minute)
    - Hip flexor stretch (1 minute)
    - Shoulder stretch (1 minute)

10-Minute Quick Morning Routine

1. **Warm-up (2 minutes)**

    - Jog in place (1 minute)
    - Arm swings (1 minute)

2. **Main Circuit (6 minutes)**

    - Lunges (30 seconds)
    - Plank (30 seconds)
    - Tricep dips (30 seconds, using a chair)
    - Rest (30 seconds)
    - Repeat the circuit 2 times

3. **Cool-down (2 minutes)**

    - Gentle yoga stretch (1 minute)

    - Deep breathing and side stretch (1 minute)

Both routines are designed for quick execution but still provide a full-body workout, perfect for days when you're short on time but still want to get moving!

Incorporating exercise into your workday might seem daunting, but it's more feasible than you think. Desk exercises are a brilliant way to keep moving without leaving your workspace. Consider seated leg lifts or desk push-ups during a conference call. These little bursts of activity can improve circulation and reduce stress, helping you stay focused and alert. If you're working from home, the possibilities expand. Try multitasking—walking on a treadmill while catching up on emails, or doing calf raises while waiting for your coffee to brew. These small but effective movements can add up, ensuring that exercise is a seamless part of your daily routine.

To make quick workouts even more accessible, consider leveraging technology. Fitness tracking apps like Tabata Pro or Nike Training Club offer quick workouts tailored to your preferences and goals. They provide structure, reminders, and motivation, turning your phone into a personal trainer. For those who prefer equipment, compact, multi-purpose items like resistance bands or adjustable dumbbells can transform any space into a mini gym. These tools are easy to store and versatile, allowing you to perform a variety of exercises without bulky machines. By embracing these resources, you ensure that time-efficient workouts remain engaging and effective, no matter where you are.

Interactive Journal: Quick Workout Planner

Take a moment to plan your week of time-efficient workouts. Identify three days where you can dedicate 20 minutes to exercise. Choose a combination of HIIT, circuit training, and desk exercises that appeal to you. Use a fitness app to guide your sessions, and make a list of any equipment you might need. This planner will help you visualize how fitness can fit into your schedule, empowering you to stay active, even on the busiest days.

Identifying 3 Days for Quick Workouts Look at your upcoming week and choose three days where you can dedicate 20 minutes to exercise. Mark them below:

- **Day 1:**

- **Day 2:**

- **Day 3:**

Choosing Your Workout Focus For each of the days you've selected, plan a quick workout session that includes a combination of HIIT, circuit training, and desk exercises.

Choose the one that resonates most with your goals and preferences.

- **Day 1:** (e.g., HIIT)

- **Day 2:** (e.g., Circuit Training)

- **Day 3:** (e.g., Desk Exercises)

Using a Fitness App for Guidance What app will you use to guide your sessions? List any specific workouts or programs that you'd like to follow.

Required Equipment Do you need any equipment for your quick workout sessions (e.g., resistance bands, dumbbells, yoga mat)? List any items you'll need to ensure you're fully prepared.

Visualizing Your Week of Fitness How do you feel about fitting fitness into your busy schedule? Does this plan feel achievable? How will you stay motivated to complete each session?

Final Thoughts What steps will you take to ensure you stick to your workout plan?

Music Suggestion For motivation, try these energizing tunes:

- **For High-Intensity Workouts:** *Can't Hold Us* by Macklemore & Ryan Lewis

- **For Circuit Training:** *Uptown Funk* by Mark Ronson ft. Bruno Mars

- **For Desk Exercise Focus:** *Happy* by Pharrell Williams

Functional Fitness for Everyday Life

Functional fitness is like the secret weapon you didn't know you needed. It's all about training your body to handle real-life activities with ease and confidence. Imagine moving through your day with improved mobility and stability—picking up your kids, carrying groceries, or even just climbing stairs can feel like a breeze. This approach focuses on exercises that mimic everyday movements, improving your ability to perform daily tasks safely and efficiently. By enhancing your body's natural movements, you not only reduce the risk of injury but also build a foundation of strength and resilience.

Think of squats not just as a gym exercise, but as a way to improve your leg strength for all those times you need to lift something heavy. Planks, too, are more than just a core workout; they stabilize your entire body, supporting balance and posture. These exercises are the building blocks of functional fitness, designed to make life easier and keep you moving without pain or strain. Incorporating them into your routine doesn't require fancy equipment or hours at the gym. It's about making small, consistent efforts that pay off big in your everyday life.

Integrating functional movements into your fitness plan is straightforward and incredibly rewarding. Start by combining these exercises with your existing workouts. If you're already doing strength training, add in sets of squats and planks to enhance your regimen. Functional fitness circuits are another great option, allowing you to cycle through a series of movements that target different muscle groups. These circuits can be tailored to fit your schedule, whether you have 10 minutes or half an hour. The key is consistency, ensuring these movements become second nature, seamlessly supporting your day-to-day activities.

The real magic of functional fitness lies in its practical applications. Imagine carrying a week's worth of groceries from the car to the kitchen without needing a break. Or think about how much easier it would be to bend and lift safely when tidying up your living space. These are the everyday victories that functional fitness delivers. It's about preparing your body for whatever life throws your way, ensuring you're ready to tackle tasks with strength and ease. As you build functional strength, you'll notice a newfound confidence in your movements, empowering you to live a more active and engaged life.

Functional fitness isn't just about exercise; it's about enhancing your quality of life. By focusing on movements that replicate real-world activities, you're training your body to be stronger and more resilient. This approach not only supports physical health but also boosts mental well-being, as the confidence gained from functional strength spills over into other areas of your life. Whether you're a busy parent, a dedicated professional, or an active retiree, functional fitness offers benefits that resonate across all aspects of your daily routine. Embrace these movements, and watch as they transform not only your body but also your approach to each day.

Low-Impact Exercises for All Ages

Imagine stepping into a world of movement that welcomes everyone, no matter your age or fitness level. Low-impact exercises are your gateway to a healthier lifestyle, offering a gentle yet effective way to stay active. These exercises are a boon for many reasons, starting with their reduced risk of injury. They are designed to be joint-friendly, making them ideal for those who want to keep moving without the strain that high-impact activities might cause. Whether you're recovering from an injury or simply looking for a more sustainable approach to fitness, low-impact exercises provide a safe space to move your body without fear of overdoing it. Their accessibility makes them an excellent choice for a wide range of individuals, from beginners just starting their fitness journey to seasoned athletes looking for a lighter workout.

Let's explore some of the low-impact exercises that can make a difference in your routine. Water aerobics is a wonderful option that combines resistance and support, making it perfect for those with joint concerns. The water cushions your movements, reducing stress on the joints while still providing a challenging workout. Another fantastic choice is walking. Often underestimated, walking is a powerful cardiovascular exercise that can be tailored to your pace and environment. Whether you're strolling through your neighborhood or hiking a scenic trail, walking offers numerous health benefits without the wear and tear of more intense workouts. These exercises are not only effective but also adaptable, allowing you to adjust the intensity and duration to match your needs and preferences.

Certain groups can particularly benefit from incorporating low-impact workouts into their lives. Seniors, for instance, may find these exercises crucial for maintaining mobility and independence. As we age, our bodies naturally lose some of their flexibility and strength, but regular low-impact exercise can counteract these changes, helping seniors stay active and engaged in daily activities. Beginners, too, can find solace in low-impact workouts as they ease into a new exercise routine. Starting with gentle movements allows them to build confidence and stamina, paving the way for more challenging activities down the line. These exercises create a foundation of fitness that supports long-term health and well-being, making them an essential component of any comprehensive fitness plan.

Incorporating low-impact exercises into your routine can be both simple and rewarding. Start by scheduling regular walking sessions into your week. Set aside time each day to step outside and enjoy a walk, even if it's just for ten minutes. Walking not only boosts cardiovascular health but also provides a mental reset, helping you clear your mind and reduce stress. Joining a community class or group can also enhance your experience. Many community centers offer classes like yoga or tai chi, which focus on gentle, flowing movements. These classes provide a supportive environment where you can learn and grow with others, fostering a sense of camaraderie and motivation. Additionally, consider exploring local resources such as parks or trails that encourage outdoor activities. These natural settings can inspire you to move more, turning exercise into an enjoyable part of your day.

Incorporating Yoga and Stretching for Flexibility

Imagine rolling out your yoga mat after a long day, the gentle hum of music in the background, as you start to unwind. Yoga is more than just a series of poses; it's a practice that invites you to extend beyond the limits of your physical body and into a space of mental clarity. This ancient practice opens doors to a deeper connection with yourself, promoting flexibility not only in muscles but in the mind as well. By engaging in yoga, you allow your body to stretch and strengthen, improving your range of motion and reducing the risk of injury in other activities. The beauty of yoga is that it meets you where you are, allowing you to progress at your own pace, fostering both patience and perseverance.

Stress reduction is one of yoga's most celebrated benefits. As you move through each pose, focusing on your breath and body, you enter a meditative state that calms the nervous system. This practice not only relaxes the mind but also releases physical tension stored in your muscles. Over time, regular yoga can lead to significant improvements in stress management, helping you cope with the demands of daily life with more ease and grace. One of the key elements of yoga is its ability to enhance flexibility. Through a consistent practice, you gradually increase your range of motion, enabling your body to move more freely. This increased flexibility supports everyday activities, reducing the likelihood of strains or sprains.

For those new to yoga, starting with basic poses can provide a solid foundation. Downward Dog is a staple, offering a full-body stretch that engages multiple muscle groups. This pose not only stretches your hamstrings and calves but also strengthens your arms and shoulders. Child's Pose, on the other hand, is a gentle resting position that encourages relaxation and introspection. It's a moment to pause, breathe, and reconnect with yourself amidst the bustle of life. These poses are accessible to beginners, offering a wonderful introduction to the benefits of yoga. Incorporating them into your routine can transform a hectic day into a peaceful retreat, leaving you refreshed and grounded.

Stretching, while often overlooked, plays a crucial role in maintaining a healthy body. Regular stretching prevents injuries by preparing your muscles for the demands of exercise and daily activities. Dynamic stretches, in particular, are excellent for pre-workout warm-ups, as they increase blood flow and enhance muscle elasticity. By incorporating stretches into your routine, you improve your overall performance, allowing your body to move with greater efficiency and power. Stretching also promotes better posture, reducing the risk of discomfort associated with long periods of sitting or standing. It's a simple yet effective way to support your body's health, ensuring you can enjoy an active lifestyle for years to come.

Creating a personalized stretching routine is a straightforward process. Begin by identifying areas of your body that feel tight or restricted. This awareness allows you to tailor your routine to address specific needs, enhancing its effectiveness. Incorporate stretches into your daily life, perhaps as part of your morning ritual or evening wind-down. Using props like yoga blocks or straps can enhance your stretching, providing support and deepening your practice. These tools are particularly useful for beginners, helping you maintain proper alignment and prevent injury. As you develop your routine, listen to your body, adjusting the intensity and duration of stretches based on how you feel each day. This flexibility ensures that your practice remains enjoyable and beneficial, supporting both your physical and mental well-being.

Strength Training for Beginners

Standing in front of a set of dumbbells, you might feel a mix of apprehension and excitement about the strength training ahead. It's more than just lifting weights—it's a gateway to building muscle, toning your body, and boosting your metabolism. Engaging in strength training can help you burn calories more efficiently, even when you're at rest. This happens because muscle tissue burns more calories than fat tissue, leading to a revved-up metabolism. It's like giving your body an engine upgrade, making it more efficient at burning fuel. Strength training also brings a sense of empowerment, as you witness your body becoming stronger and more capable, which can boost confidence and well-being.

Let's address some common misconceptions that might hold you back. One of the biggest myths is the fear of becoming too bulky, especially for women. The reality is, building substantial muscle mass requires specific training and dietary conditions. Most strength training routines will result in a toned physique rather than bulk. Another misunderstanding is the assumption that weight lifting is solely about aesthetics. In truth, it offers a plethora of benefits beyond appearance, such as improved bone density, better balance, and enhanced mental health. These myths can deter beginners, but understanding the real benefits can inspire you to incorporate strength training into your routine with confidence.

For those new to strength training, starting with bodyweight exercises is a fantastic way to ease into it. Exercises like push-ups and lunges are effective in building foundational strength without the need for equipment. These movements engage multiple muscle groups, improving overall fitness and coordination. As you become more comfortable, consider introducing resistance bands into your routine. They offer a versatile, portable option to add resistance and increase the challenge of your workouts. Resistance bands come in various tensions, allowing you to gradually increase intensity as your strength improves. This progression ensures that you continue to make gains without risking injury.

Proper form and technique are crucial in strength training to prevent injuries and maximize results. Each exercise has a specific form that ensures you're targeting the right muscles while protecting your joints and spine. For example, when performing a squat, you should keep your feet shoulder-width apart, engage your core, and ensure your knees don't extend beyond your toes. Maintaining these cues helps prevent strain and promotes muscle engagement. If you're uncertain about your form, consider using resources like online tutorials, fitness apps, or even a session with a personal trainer. These tools can provide guidance and feedback, helping you learn the correct techniques and build confidence in your abilities.

As you incorporate strength training into your fitness plan, remember that consistency is key. Gradually increase the intensity and complexity of your workouts as your body adapts. Listen to your body, allowing time for rest and recovery, which are just as important as the workouts themselves. By doing so, you'll create a balanced approach that supports long-term health and fitness goals. Embrace the journey of strength training with curiosity and patience, knowing that each session brings you closer to a stronger, healthier you.

Strength training is a powerful component of a well-rounded fitness routine, offering benefits that extend beyond the physical. It supports mental resilience, fosters discipline, and cultivates a sense of accomplishment. As you conclude this chapter, reflect on how the principles of personalized fitness, time-efficient workouts, functional movements, low-impact exercises, yoga, and finally, strength training, can come together to create a lifestyle that suits you. Each element plays a role in supporting your well-being, paving the way for a healthier, more vibrant life. As we transition to the next chapter, prepare to explore how these practices can be woven into daily routines, making wellness an integral part of who you are.

Chapter 4

Creating Lasting Habits

Waking up to the first light of dawn, you reach for your running shoes, not out of obligation, but because it's the best way to kickstart your day. Habits, those intricate patterns we weave into our lives, can be both our allies and our adversaries. They are the silent architects shaping our daily routines and, ultimately, our lives. Understanding how habits form is like holding the blueprint to change—we can redesign our behaviors, one brick at a time. At the heart of this transformation lies the basal ganglia, a deep-set cluster of brain structures responsible for habit memory. This region orchestrates the automatic behaviors that make up the fabric of our lives, evolving simple actions into habits through repeated practice. Habits form through a loop: a trigger prompts a routine, which leads to a reward. This cycle becomes ingrained over time, making actions second nature and freeing our minds to focus on more complex tasks.

The beauty of habits lies in their ability to grow from tiny seeds into towering oaks. The power of tiny changes, or what I like to call the 1% improvement principle, demonstrates how small, incremental adjustments can lead to profound changes over time. This concept underscores that you don't need massive leaps to make progress; instead, aim for steady, consistent growth. Imagine improving by just 1% each day. While it may seem insignificant, over the course of a year, these small changes compound, making you substantially better. This approach is less daunting than overhauling your entire routine at once, which often leads to burnout. Instead, focus on making manageable tweaks that align with your goals and lifestyle, gradually building momentum and confidence. This philosophy champions patience and persistence, reminding us that sustainable change happens over time, not overnight.

Consistency is the lifeblood of habit formation. It's the daily repetition, the showing up even when you don't feel like it, that solidifies new behaviors into habits. Like a craftsman honing their skills, it's the regular practice that refines and perfects. Missing a day isn't the end of the world, but it can disrupt the rhythm you've worked hard to establish. Think of habit building like tending to a garden; it requires consistent care and attention. Skipping a day might not ruin your progress, but it does highlight the importance of returning to your routine as soon as possible. Consistency builds trust in yourself, reinforcing the belief that you can rely on your habits to guide you through life's challenges. It's about creating a chain of positive actions, where each link strengthens the next, until your new habit feels as natural as breathing.

Aligning habits with your identity is a powerful way to strengthen your commitment. This concept, known as habit identity, suggests that when you see your habits as part of who you are, they become more deeply ingrained. Instead of saying, "I want to exercise more," shift your mindset to "I am someone who exercises regularly." This subtle change in language shifts your perception, aligning your actions with your identity. When your habits reflect your self-image, you're more likely to stick with them, as they become an expression of who you are. This alignment between habits and identity creates a sense of authenticity and purpose, motivating you to maintain your new behaviors. Consider athletes who identify as disciplined; their training becomes a natural extension of their identity, not just a means to an end. By embedding your habits into your self-concept, you create a powerful framework for lasting change.

<u>Reflection Journal</u>

Take a moment to reflect on a habit you wish to cultivate. Write down how this habit aligns with your identity and values. Consider how adopting this habit can reinforce your self-image and contribute to your personal growth. What small changes can you implement today to start aligning your actions with *this new identity? Use this reflection as a guide to help you integrate your habits into the fabric of who you are, creating a path towards positive transformation.*

Reflecting on a Habit I Wish to Cultivate Take a moment to think about a habit you wish to cultivate. How does this habit align with your identity and core values? Why is it important to you?

Connecting the Habit to My Self-Image How will adopting this habit help reinforce your self-image and contribute to your personal growth? What aspects of your identity does this habit reflect or support?

Small Changes to Begin the Journey What small actions or changes can you implement today or this week to start aligning your actions with your new identity? How can you make these changes feel natural and achievable?

Integrating the Habit into My Life What steps will you take to ensure this habit becomes a consistent part of your life? How will you track your progress and stay motivated?

Final Thoughts How does reflecting on this habit make you feel? What impact do you hope to see by integrating this habit into your daily routine?

Music Suggestion Pair your reflection with music that helps you focus and feel empowered:

- **For Calm and Clarity:** *Weightless* by Marconi Union

- **For Motivation and Focus:** *Rise Up* by Andra Day

- **For Positive Vibes:** *Good as Hell* by Lizzo

Habit Stacking for Seamless Integration

Ever find yourself brushing your teeth and wondering if there's a way to maximize those two minutes? That's where habit stacking comes in. It's a clever strategy that makes it easier to form new habits by linking them to existing ones. Essentially, habit stacking uses your current routines as a springboard for developing new behaviors. The idea is simple: by tacking a new habit onto an already established one, you create a sequence that feels natural and effortless. This way, the established habit acts as a trigger for the new one, making it more likely to stick.

To create a habit stack, start by identifying the daily routines that are already part of your life. These can be anything from making your morning coffee to locking the front door as you leave for work. These routines serve as anchors, providing a stable foundation for your new habits. For example, if you're looking to incorporate meditation into your day, consider adding it right after you pour your morning coffee. This way, the act of brewing coffee becomes a signal to meditate. Similarly, if you want to stretch more often, link it to brushing your teeth. As you finish brushing, use that moment to engage in a quick stretch. By associating new habits with existing ones, you sidestep the need to carve out additional time or create a new routine from scratch.

Habit stacking shines in real-world applications. Consider how you can transform your busy mornings. Perhaps you want to start expressing gratitude each day. Simply stack this new habit onto your existing routine of sitting down for breakfast. As your cereal bowl hits the table, take a moment to reflect on one thing you're thankful for. Or imagine integrating a brief workout into your evening. As soon as you change into your comfortable clothes after work, do a quick set of squats. These stacks blend seamlessly into your life, turning potential obstacles into opportunities. By piggybacking on habits you already perform, you reduce the mental load of decision-making, making it easier to adopt new behaviors.

One of the greatest benefits of habit stacking is its ability to simplify habit formation, especially for those of us juggling multiple responsibilities. By reducing decision fatigue, habit stacking streamlines your day, allowing you to focus on what truly matters. Decision fatigue occurs when you're faced with too many choices, leading to exhaustion and poor decision-making. By pre-determining when and where you'll perform a new habit, you eliminate the need for constant decision-making, freeing up mental energy. This efficiency not only makes it easier to incorporate new habits but also enhances your overall productivity and well-being.

Habit stacking is like building a chain of events, where each link is a habit that leads seamlessly into the next. This method leverages the power of routine, making new habits feel as automatic as brushing your teeth or drinking your morning coffee. Over time, these stacked habits create a ripple effect, improving various aspects of your life without overwhelming you with change. As you experiment with different habit stacks, you'll uncover a rhythm that works for you, one that aligns with your lifestyle and values. The beauty of habit stacking lies in its simplicity and adaptability, making it a versatile tool for anyone seeking to enhance their daily routine.

Overcoming Barriers to Change

We've all been there: feeling like there aren't enough hours in the day to fit in something new. One of the most common barriers to forming new habits is a lack of time. Between work, family, and personal commitments, it can seem impossible to squeeze in anything extra, even if it's beneficial. Time management becomes crucial here. Think of your schedule as a puzzle, where every piece needs to fit just right. Start by evaluating your daily routines and identifying pockets of time that can be repurposed. Perhaps it's those 15 minutes after dinner or the quiet moments before everyone else wakes up. Use these snippets wisely, turning them into opportunities for growth.

Another formidable barrier is the fear of failure. It's that little voice that whispers doubts, making you hesitate before trying something new. Yet, failure isn't the end; it's a stepping stone to learning. Reframing failure as a learning opportunity can shift your perspective. Each setback is a chance to gather insights and refine your approach. Embrace the idea that mistakes are part of the process, not a judgment of your worth. By adopting a growth mindset, you open yourself up to possibilities, seeing each attempt as progress, regardless of the outcome. This mindset encourages resilience, allowing you to bounce back stronger after each stumble.

Let's talk about environment design, a powerful yet often overlooked tool for facilitating habit change. Your surroundings influence your behavior more than you might realize. By creating physical cues for your habits, you make them more visible and accessible. For instance, if you're trying to drink more water, place a water bottle on your desk as a constant reminder. Reducing friction for positive behaviors is another effective strategy. Make the desired actions easy to start and hard to ignore. Set out your workout clothes the night before, or prep healthy snacks at eye level in the fridge. These small tweaks can significantly increase the likelihood of following through with your intentions.

On the flip side, let's address the psychological barriers that often come with change. Overcoming resistance requires mental strategies that enhance your resilience. Visualization is a powerful tool here. Picture yourself successfully adopting the new habit, feeling the emotions of accomplishment and satisfaction. This mental rehearsal primes your mind for success, making the actual process feel more natural. Self-affirmation practices can also bolster your resolve. By regularly reminding yourself of your strengths and capabilities, you build confidence in your ability to change. Write down affirmations that resonate with you and repeat them daily. They serve as a gentle nudge, encouraging you to persevere even when the going gets tough.

These strategies are your allies in the quest to overcome barriers to change. They remind you that while obstacles are real, they are not insurmountable. With a little creativity and determination, you can navigate these challenges, turning them into stepping stones on your path to personal growth and self-care.

Setting Realistic and Achievable Goals

Starting a new fitness plan or adopting healthier eating habits often begins with enthusiasm and energy. However, a common challenge arises when goals are set too ambitiously or vaguely, leading to feelings of overwhelm or uncertainty. That's where the magic of realistic goal setting comes into play. It's about crafting goals that motivate you without overwhelming, goals that are clear and achievable. This approach is crucial because it keeps you on track and builds confidence as you achieve each milestone. Enter the WISE goals framework—an approach that ensures your goals are Worthwhile, Inspiring, Specific, and Evaluated. Worthwhile means your goals should align with your values and passions, making them personally meaningful. Inspiring should spark motivation, pushing you towards action. Specific goals are clear and detailed, leaving no room for ambiguity. Lastly, goals should be Evaluated regularly, allowing you to track progress and adjust as needed. With this framework, you can create goals that not only inspire but also guide you towards success.

The process of setting goals is like mapping out a journey. It starts with defining what you want to achieve, breaking it down into manageable steps. This step-by-step approach turns a daunting task into a series of achievable actions, making progress feel natural and attainable. Let's say your goal is to improve your fitness. Begin by outlining small, specific actions, such as committing to a 15-minute walk each day. As you build confidence, gradually increase the intensity or duration of your walks. Setting timelines for accountability is another essential aspect of this process. Timelines provide structure, creating a sense of urgency that keeps you focused and motivated. Consider setting both short-term and long-term timelines, allowing you to celebrate small victories while staying committed to your larger goals. This structured approach ensures that your goals remain both realistic and within reach, paving the way for sustainable change.

Flexibility is the unsung hero of goal setting. As you pursue your goals, life happens—unexpected challenges arise or priorities shift. That's why it's essential to approach goals with a flexible mindset. Flexibility allows you to adapt and adjust your goals as needed, without feeling like you're abandoning them. It's about understanding that progress isn't always linear, and that's okay. Imagine you've set a goal to work out every morning, but suddenly, your schedule changes due to work commitments. Instead of giving up, adjust your goal to fit your new routine—perhaps working out in the evenings or finding shorter, more intense workouts. This adaptability keeps your goals relevant and achievable, even in the face of change. It encourages resilience, reminding you that setbacks are not failures but opportunities to reassess and refocus.

The beauty of setting realistic and achievable goals lies in the empowerment it brings. As you accomplish each step, your confidence grows, reinforcing your belief in your ability to achieve more. This positive reinforcement creates a cycle of success, where each achievement propels you towards the next goal. It's about building momentum, where the satisfaction of progress fuels your motivation. As you continue to refine your goals, remember to celebrate your achievements, no matter how small they may seem. Each victory is a testament to your dedication and perseverance, a reminder that you're capable of achieving great things. Whether you're striving for better health, personal growth, or professional success, setting realistic goals provides a clear path forward, guiding you closer to the life you envision.

Maintaining Motivation Through Accountability

Starting a new fitness program often begins with high spirits and enthusiasm, but as time progresses, this initial zeal can sometimes diminish, a scenario many find familiar. It's during these moments that the concept of accountability becomes indispensable, serving as a crucial bridge to sustain your commitment. Far from being just a trendy term, accountability emerges as a significant driving force that strengthens your determination to persevere. The benefits of partnering with a workout buddy or an accountability partner are profound. Such partners act as your cheerleader and motivator, applauding your achievements and providing that gentle push when your drive starts to falter. Whether it's a close friend, a family member, or a work colleague, their involvement in your fitness journey can significantly amplify your motivation. The knowledge that you have someone rooting for your success can be tremendously supportive, helping to either preserve or even elevate the enthusiasm you had at the outset.

Building accountability structures can be as simple or as elaborate as you like. Joining health and wellness groups, whether online or in your community, is a fantastic way to surround yourself with like-minded individuals who share your goals. These groups offer a sense of camaraderie and mutual motivation, turning individual efforts into a collective journey. Social media can also be a surprisingly effective tool for public commitment. By sharing your goals and progress with your online network, you create a layer of accountability that's both personal and public. The likes, comments, and encouragement you receive can be incredibly motivating, reinforcing your commitment to your goals. Plus, by putting your intentions out there, you create a sense of responsibility to follow through, knowing others are rooting for you.

Tracking progress is another cornerstone of maintaining motivation. It's one thing to set goals, but monitoring your journey provides tangible evidence of your efforts. Visual progress charts, whether digital or on paper, offer a clear view of how far you've come. They transform abstract goals into concrete achievements, providing a snapshot of your progress at a glance. This visual representation serves as a reminder that every small step counts, each effort adding to the bigger picture of success. Seeing your achievements mapped out can reignite motivation, especially on days when you might question your progress. Tracking allows you to celebrate milestones, big or small, reinforcing your dedication and propelling you forward.

The psychological impact of accountability cannot be overstated. Social reinforcement plays a crucial role in shaping behaviors, as we often adjust our actions based on the expectations and support of those around us. The knowledge that others are aware of your goals can create a sense of responsibility, motivating you to stay on track. Additionally, there's a psychological motivator that comes from the fear of disappointing others. While it's not about seeking external validation, the desire to meet the expectations of those cheering you on can be a powerful incentive. Knowing that someone else believes in your potential can bolster your own self-belief, encouraging you to push through challenges and persevere.

Accountability is about creating a support system that fosters resilience and commitment. It's the safety net that catches you when motivation wavers, offering encouragement and guidance to keep you on course. Whether it's through peer support, structured groups, or personal tracking, accountability provides a framework for success. It transforms solitary efforts into a shared experience, where each step forward is celebrated and supported. As you explore different ways to incorporate accountability into your routine, remember that it's a dynamic process, one that evolves alongside your goals and aspirations. Embrace the connections and structures that resonate with you, knowing they are allies in your pursuit of lasting change.

Tracking Progress and Celebrating Milestones

Imagine setting off on a new fitness routine or dietary change, filled with motivation and hope. As the days roll by, it's easy to lose sight of the progress you're making. This is where tracking progress becomes not just helpful but transformative. It's like looking in the mirror and seeing the subtle changes that might otherwise go unnoticed. Tracking provides a snapshot of where you started, where you are, and where you're headed. By recording daily habits, you create a log that captures each step forward. Whether it's noting the days you exercised, the meals you prepared, or the moments you practiced mindfulness, these entries serve as a tangible reflection of your efforts. Over time, analyzing trends helps you identify patterns—what works, what doesn't, and how you can fine-tune your approach for even better results.

The joy of reaching a milestone, no matter how small, is immense. Celebrating these moments is not just about the satisfaction of accomplishment, but about reinforcing your commitment and boosting your morale. It's like giving yourself a little pat on the back for a job well done. Planning small rewards for hitting these milestones can be incredibly motivating. Maybe it's a new book you've been eyeing, a relaxing spa day, or a simple afternoon off to enjoy your favorite hobby. These rewards don't have to be extravagant; they just need to be meaningful to you. Reflection on your progress to date is equally important. Taking the time to look back at what you've achieved can reignite your motivation and remind you why you started. It's about acknowledging the effort and dedication you've invested, which fuels the drive to keep going.

To effectively track your progress, consider using tools that fit seamlessly into your lifestyle. Habit tracking apps are a convenient option, offering a digital platform to log your activities and visualize your progress. These apps often come with reminders and customizable features, making it easy to stay on top of your goals. If you prefer a more tactile approach, bullet journaling techniques offer a creative and personalized way to track your journey. With a bullet journal, you can design layouts that suit your needs, incorporating habit trackers, mood logs, and reflection pages. This method allows for flexibility and creativity, turning progress tracking into a rewarding and artistic endeavor.

Reflection plays a crucial role in the development of positive habits. Regular review sessions create a space for introspection, allowing you to assess what's working and what needs adjustment. By setting aside time to reflect, you reinforce the habits you're cultivating, making them more ingrained in your daily routine. This process also highlights areas where you might need to adapt your strategies. Perhaps a certain habit isn't aligning with your schedule as well as you'd hoped, or maybe you've discovered a new approach that yields better results. Being open to change and willing to adjust your plan based on these reflections is key to long-term success.

In tracking your progress and celebrating your milestones, you create a roadmap of your journey towards holistic wellness. Each entry, each reflection, and each celebration contributes to a deeper understanding of yourself and your capabilities. As you continue to build on these habits, you're not just working towards a goal—you're transforming your lifestyle. This chapter serves as a reminder that every step, no matter how small, is a step forward. As you embrace this mindset, you'll find that the path to wellness is not about perfection but progress. In the next chapter, we'll explore how mindful living and stress management can further enhance your well-being, providing you with tools to navigate life's challenges with grace and resilience.

Chapter 5

Mindful Living and Stress Management

Stress seems to be the unwelcome guest that sneaks into your life when you least expect it. Maybe it's a looming work deadline or a tense conversation with a family member that sets your heart racing and your mind spiraling. Stress triggers are the culprits behind this all-too-familiar feeling. They are specific events or situations that provoke a stress response, and they vary widely from person to person. Identifying these triggers is crucial for managing stress effectively. By understanding what sets off your stress response, you can start to develop strategies to mitigate its impact, transforming stress from an overpowering force into a manageable part of life.

Common stress triggers often revolve around the demands of work and family. Picture this: you're juggling a pile of tasks at work, and just as you're about to make headway, an email pops up with a new deadline. Your heart rate quickens, hands get clammy, and suddenly, you're overwhelmed. Family conflicts can be another trigger, whether it's a disagreement over parenting styles or managing household responsibilities. These situations can escalate quickly, leading to a familiar knot in your stomach. Recognizing these triggers helps in understanding the physiological and emotional responses that follow. Stress isn't just in your head; it manifests physically. An increased heart rate, shallow breathing, and a flood of anxiety are telltale signs. Over time, unchecked stress can lead to chronic fatigue, weaken your immune system, and make you more susceptible to illnesses.

Identifying your unique stressors starts with self-reflection and observation. Keeping a stress diary can be an invaluable tool. Note down situations that trigger stress, your emotional and physical responses, and any patterns you notice. Over time, this journal becomes a map of your stress landscape, revealing consistent triggers and helping you anticipate them. Reflective questioning techniques can also be enlightening. Ask yourself what exactly about a situation causes stress. Is it the fear of failure, the pressure of time, or perhaps a lack of control? Understanding these nuances allows you to address the root causes, rather than just the symptoms.

Once you've identified your stress triggers, it's time to develop strategies to manage your responses. Cognitive behavioral techniques can be particularly effective. These methods encourage you to challenge and change negative thought patterns, replacing them with more balanced perspectives. For example, if a work deadline causes stress, instead of thinking, "I'll never finish," try reframing it to, "I'll tackle this one step at a time." Developing coping mechanisms is another key strategy. This might involve engaging in activities that naturally reduce stress, such as exercise, creative pursuits, or spending time in nature. These activities provide a healthy outlet for stress, allowing you to process emotions and return to a state of calm.

Stress Management Journal Prompt

Take a moment to write about a recent situation that triggered stress. Describe the event, your immediate reactions, and how you managed it. Reflect on what you could do differently next time. Consider how cognitive behavioral techniques could alter your perspective or how a new coping strategy might ease your response. This exercise is a step toward proactive stress management, empowering you to navigate life's challenges with resilience and clarity.

Reflecting on a Recent Stressful Situation Take a moment to write about a recent situation that triggered stress. What happened? How did you feel in the moment, and what were your immediate reactions?

How I Managed the Stress How did you manage the situation? Did you use any coping strategies or stress-relief techniques in the moment? How effective were they?

What I Could Do Differently Looking back, what could you have done differently to manage your stress more effectively? Were there any thoughts or behaviors that contributed to the stress response that you could adjust?

Incorporating Cognitive Behavioral Techniques How could cognitive behavioral techniques (such as reframing thoughts, identifying cognitive distortions, or challenging negative beliefs) help you respond differently in the future?

New Coping Strategies for Future Stress What new coping strategies could you implement the next time you encounter stress? Consider relaxation techniques, mindfulness practices, or healthier responses.

Final Thoughts How do you feel about your approach to stress management after reflecting on this situation? What will you do moving forward to build resilience and clarity in challenging moments?

Music Suggestion Pair this reflection with calming music to encourage relaxation:

- **For Relaxation and Focus:** *Weightless* by Marconi Union

- **For Stress Relief:** *Sunset Lover* by Petit Biscuit

- **For Positive Energy:** *Don't Stop Believin'* by Journey

Mindfulness Techniques for Stress Relief

Standing at the edge of a serene lake, with its calm and reflective waters, evokes a sense of stillness. Mindfulness is akin to this stillness—a tool that brings clarity and peace amidst life's turbulence. It's about focusing on the present moment, tuning into the here and now rather than getting lost in the whirlwind of past regrets or future anxieties. Mindfulness can significantly reduce stress by drawing your attention away from the chaos and back to your breath, your body, and your immediate surroundings. This practice doesn't just calm the mind; it grounds you, helping you navigate life with a steady heart and an open mind.

There are various mindfulness practices that you can explore, each offering a unique path to stress relief. One gentle and compassionate technique is Loving Kindness meditation. This practice involves silently repeating phrases of goodwill and encouragement, first directed towards yourself and then extended to others. By fostering feelings of love and connection, you cultivate a sense of peace, which can be a balm for stress. Mindful Movement is another wonderful practice. Whether it's yoga, tai chi, or simply walking, moving mindfully involves paying attention to each movement, each breath, allowing you to become fully immersed in the experience. Lastly, there's Body Scanning, where you mentally scan your body from head to toe, noticing areas of tension and relaxation, without judgment. This technique fosters a deep sense of body awareness, helping to release stress and enhance relaxation.

The benefits of regular mindfulness practice go beyond immediate stress relief. Over time, mindfulness can increase your resilience to stress, allowing you to handle life's challenges with greater ease. It helps improve emotional regulation, giving you the tools to respond thoughtfully rather than react impulsively to stressful situations. Regular mindfulness practice can also lead to enhanced concentration and emotional stability, supporting overall well-being. As you cultivate mindfulness, you may find that you're more present in your interactions, more attuned to your emotions, and more capable of maintaining balance in the face of adversity.

Starting a mindfulness practice doesn't require a major overhaul of your daily routine. It's about setting aside a few moments each day to be present with yourself. Begin by choosing a time that suits you, whether it's in the morning to set the tone for the day or in the evening to unwind. Find a quiet space where you won't be disturbed, and sit comfortably, closing your eyes if you wish. Start with a few deep breaths, allowing your mind to settle. You might choose to focus on your breathing, noting each inhale and exhale, or you might prefer a guided mindfulness resource, such as a meditation app or online video. These resources can provide structure and guidance, especially as you're starting out. Remember, mindfulness is a skill that develops over time with practice and dedication, so be patient and kind to yourself as you explore this transformative practice.

The Power of Meditation in Daily Life

Picture yourself sitting comfortably, eyes gently closed, as the chaos of the day fades into the background. This is the transformative power of meditation—a practice that not only calms the mind but also rejuvenates the spirit. Meditation serves as a powerful tool in stress management, primarily by its ability to reduce cortisol levels, the hormone that rises during stressful situations. By lowering cortisol, meditation helps alleviate stress, promoting a sense of calm and mental clarity. It's like giving your mind a much-needed rest, allowing you to approach life with renewed focus and energy.

When it comes to meditation, there's no one-size-fits-all approach. Different styles cater to various preferences, making it accessible to everyone. Transcendental meditation, for example, involves repeating a specific mantra to help settle the mind into a state of profound rest. This technique can be incredibly relaxing, providing an escape from the relentless pace of everyday life. Loving-kindness meditation, on the other hand, focuses on cultivating compassion and love towards oneself and others. It encourages you to foster positive emotions, which can have a ripple effect on your mental well-being. Guided imagery is another powerful form, where you visualize calming and peaceful scenes, helping to ease tension and promote relaxation. Each style offers unique benefits, allowing you to choose what resonates most with your needs and lifestyle.

The impact of meditation on mental health is profound. Regular practice enhances focus and concentration, sharpening your mind and enabling you to tackle tasks with greater efficiency. It's like exercising your brain, building the muscle of attention and presence. Moreover, meditation is known to improve mood, fostering positive emotions and reducing feelings of anxiety and depression. Through meditation, you create a space for self-reflection and acceptance, nurturing a healthier relationship with your thoughts and emotions. This practice empowers you to let go of negativity, embracing a more balanced and harmonious state of mind.

Incorporating meditation into your daily routine doesn't have to be a daunting task. Start by scheduling it like you would any other important appointment or class. Set aside a few minutes each day, perhaps in the morning to center yourself before the day begins, or in the evening to unwind and reflect. Consistency is key, even if it's just five minutes a day. When you find yourself overwhelmed by life's demands, take a break to meditate instead of pushing through. This pause can be incredibly refreshing, offering a moment to reset and regain composure. As you explore meditation, remember that it's a personal journey. Be patient and compassionate with yourself as you discover the style and routine that best supports your well-being.

Prioritizing Sleep for Optimal Health

Ever notice how everything feels a bit more overwhelming after a sleepless night? That's because sleep plays a crucial role in managing stress and maintaining emotional balance. When you get enough sleep, your brain has the chance to process emotions and memories, which helps regulate mood and stress levels. It's like hitting the reset button, giving your mind and body a fresh start each day. Without adequate sleep, you might find yourself more irritable and less able to cope with life's challenges. Sleep is not just about resting your body; it's about rejuvenating your mind and preparing yourself to handle whatever comes your way.

Improving your sleep quality can make a world of difference, and it starts with a consistent sleep schedule. Going to bed and waking up at the same time each day, even on weekends, helps regulate your body's internal clock, making it easier to fall asleep and wake up naturally. Creating a restful sleep environment is just as important. Think of your bedroom as a sanctuary—cool, quiet, and dark. Consider investing in blackout curtains, or use a sleep mask to keep out unwanted light. A white noise machine or fan can help drown out disruptive sounds. It's all about crafting a space that invites relaxation and supports deep, restorative sleep.

Sleep hygiene refers to the practices that promote better sleep, and it's an integral part of achieving restful nights. Limiting screen time before bed is a biggie. The blue light emitted by phones, tablets, and computers can interfere with the production of melatonin, the hormone that regulates sleep. Try to power down electronics at least an hour before bedtime. Instead, engage in relaxing activities like reading a book, taking a warm bath, or practicing gentle stretches.

These routines signal your body that it's time to wind down, easing the transition into sleep.

Restorative sleep offers a treasure trove of benefits, enhancing both physical and mental health. When you sleep well, your cognitive function improves, making it easier to concentrate, remember details, and solve problems. You might find that your mind feels sharper, and tasks that once seemed daunting become more manageable. Quality sleep also boosts your immune system. During sleep, your body produces cytokines, proteins that help fight infection and inflammation. Adequate rest gives your body the strength it needs to fend off illnesses, keeping you healthier in the long run.

Digital Detox: Reclaiming Your Mind for Mindfulness

In today's hyperconnected world, the relentless influx of notifications, emails, and social media updates can leave us feeling overwhelmed and stressed. This digital overload not only affects our mental well-being but also hampers our ability to focus and be present. A digital detox offers a refreshing pause from constant connectivity, allowing you to reclaim your time and mental space. By consciously reducing screen time, you create room for mindfulness and self-care, fostering a healthier and more intentional relationship with technology.

The Impact of Digital Overload

Constant connectivity often leads to social media comparisons and information overload, both of which contribute to heightened stress and anxiety. Scrolling through curated feeds can trigger feelings of inadequacy or FOMO (fear of missing out), while the endless barrage of news and updates can leave you feeling anxious and mentally exhausted. The pressure to keep up with this digital deluge often pulls us away from meaningful, real-world experiences.

The Benefits of a Digital Detox

Taking intentional breaks from digital devices can significantly enhance your overall well-being. Disconnecting improves sleep quality by reducing late-night disruptions from notifications and limiting the temptation to stay up scrolling. This practice supports your body's natural sleep rhythms, leading to more restful nights and energized mornings.

A digital detox also strengthens interpersonal relationships by encouraging face-to-face communication. With fewer digital distractions, you can engage more deeply with loved ones, fostering connection and understanding. By stepping away from screens, you create space for meaningful conversations, shared experiences, and genuine presence.

Practical Steps for a Digital Detox

Embarking on a digital detox doesn't mean severing ties with technology altogether. Instead, it's about finding a balance that works for you. Start by setting specific times for device use. For example, designate tech-free periods during meals or an hour before bedtime. Creating boundaries protects your mental space and encourages you to engage more fully with your surroundings.

Consider designating tech-free zones in your home, such as the dining room or bedroom, to promote device-free interactions and rest. Engage in screen-free activities to rediscover hobbies or interests that bring you joy. Whether it's reading a physical book, going for a walk, painting, or gardening, these activities enrich your life and provide opportunities for relaxation and personal growth.

Reclaiming Balance and Presence

A digital detox isn't about rejecting technology but rather about reclaiming your time and attention. By consciously choosing how and when to engage with screens, you ensure that technology serves you without overwhelming you. This mindful approach creates space for moments of presence and joy that often get lost in the digital shuffle.

Imagine starting your day without your smartphone commanding your immediate attention. Instead, you take a few moments to savor the quiet or engage in a calming morning routine. By reducing your digital consumption, you relieve the burden of being perpetually online, allowing you to refocus on the tangible world and the vibrant life unfolding around you.

Whether it's the simplicity of a conversation over coffee, the quiet beauty of a sunset, or the satisfaction of completing a creative project, these moments ground you in the here and now. A digital detox helps you rediscover these experiences, enriching your life and nurturing your mental and emotional well-being.

Cultivating a Positive Mindset

Life can sometimes feel like a relentless series of challenges, each one demanding more energy and patience than the last. In these moments, a positive mindset becomes your armor against stress. It's not about pretending everything is perfect but about finding strength in optimism. Positivity acts as a buffer, helping you bounce back from adversity. When you cultivate optimism, you're essentially building resilience, making it easier to navigate life's ups and downs. Think of it as a mental muscle that, when flexed regularly, grows stronger and more robust, ready to support you through any storm.

To foster a positive mindset, consider integrating gratitude journaling into your daily routine. This practice involves jotting down things you're thankful for, no matter how small. Perhaps it's the warmth of your morning coffee or a kind word from a friend. Focusing on gratitude shifts your perspective from scarcity to abundance, reminding you of the good that exists even on tough days. Positive affirmations are another powerful tool. These are statements you repeat to yourself, such as "I am capable" or "I am worthy." They help counteract negative self-talk, reinforcing a more constructive and encouraging dialogue in your mind. By embracing these techniques, you nurture a mindset that looks for possibilities rather than problems.

Self-compassion plays a crucial role in maintaining positivity. It's about being gentle with yourself, especially when things don't go as planned. Mindful self-reflection encourages you to observe your thoughts and feelings without judgment, allowing you to understand and accept your experiences. Practicing self-forgiveness is equally important. We all make mistakes, but dwelling on them only fuels stress. Instead, acknowledge your missteps, learn from them, and let them go. This approach reduces the emotional burden you carry, promoting a healthier, more forgiving relationship with yourself.

Maintaining a positive outlook, especially during challenging times, requires conscious effort. Surrounding yourself with positive influences is a powerful strategy. Engage with people who uplift and inspire you, whether they are friends, family, or mentors. Their energy can be contagious, helping you stay motivated and optimistic. Engaging in activities that bring joy and fulfillment is equally vital. Whether it's reading, gardening, or playing an instrument, these pursuits provide an emotional boost, reminding you of the simple pleasures in life. By actively choosing positivity, you create a mental environment where stress struggles to take hold.

As you cultivate a positive mindset and integrate these practices into your life, you'll find that stress loses some of its power. You'll feel more equipped to handle whatever comes your way, with a sense of calm and clarity. This chapter has offered tools and strategies to help you navigate stress with resilience and grace. As we move forward, you'll discover how these principles can be applied to other areas of your life, building a foundation for lasting well-being.

Chapter 6

Ethical and Environmental Considerations

Picture a grocery aisle lined with an overwhelming array of food products. Each one has a story that begins on a farm and ends on your dinner table. Understanding this journey—how food travels from farm to table—is not just about knowing what you're eating, but also about recognizing the broader impacts of your choices. The processes involved in food production and distribution are complex, often hidden behind the convenience of pre-packaged goods. Transparency in the supply chain is crucial for making informed decisions. Knowing where your food comes from allows you to consider the environmental and ethical implications of its production. Industrial agriculture, for instance, plays a significant role in this narrative. While it boosts productivity to meet global demands, it also contributes to pollution through fertilizer runoff, methane emissions, and other pollutants. This is a reminder of the unseen cost of our food choices, urging us to look beyond the labels and consider the bigger picture.

When we delve into the ethical considerations of food production, the moral issues become even clearer. Fair trade practices, for example, ensure that farmers receive fair compensation for their labor, promoting sustainable livelihoods and ethical treatment. Yet, in many agricultural sectors, labor conditions remain challenging, with workers facing long hours, low wages, and sometimes unsafe environments. These conditions highlight the need for ethical consumerism—a conscious effort to support practices that prioritize human dignity and environmental stewardship. By choosing products from ethical sources, you can drive positive change in the food industry. This concept of voting with your dollars empowers you to influence the market, encouraging companies to adopt fair and sustainable practices. Supporting local farmers is another impactful choice. By buying locally, you reduce the carbon footprint associated with long-distance transportation and contribute to the vitality of your community's economy.

Navigating the grocery store aisles, you might come across various labels and certifications indicating ethical practices. These labels can guide you in making choices that align with your values. Organic certification, for instance, assures you that the product was grown without synthetic fertilizers or pesticides, supporting biodiversity and soil health. Similarly, the Fair Trade label signals that the product was made with respect for workers' rights and environmental sustainability. These certifications serve as beacons of trust, guiding you toward products that uphold ethical standards. However, not all certifications are created equal, and understanding what each represents is key to making informed decisions. Take the time to familiarize yourself with these labels, as they provide a valuable tool in your journey toward conscientious consumerism.

Interactive Journal: Ethical Shopping Checklist

Next time you shop, use this checklist to guide your choices:
   1. *Look for organic and Fair Trade certifications.*

   2. *Choose products with transparent supply chains.*

   3. *Support local farmers by buying from farmer's markets.*

   4. *Consider the environmental impact of packaging.*

By incorporating these considerations into your shopping habits, you become part of a movement towards a more ethical and sustainable food system. This shift not only benefits the planet but also fosters a deeper connection with the food you consume, enhancing your overall well-being and supporting a *future where ethical and environmental considerations are at the forefront of our choices.*

Navigating Plant-Based Nutrition

Imagine your plate filled with vibrant colors—greens, reds, yellows—all promising not only nourishment but also a healthier planet. Plant-based diets have gained attention for their numerous benefits, and with good reason. Reducing meat consumption can significantly lower the risk of chronic diseases such as heart disease, diabetes, and certain cancers. Studies have shown that a diet rich in fruits, vegetables, whole grains, and legumes can improve overall health and longevity. But the advantages extend beyond personal health. Shifting towards plant-based eating also means a reduced carbon footprint. Meat production, particularly beef, is a major contributor to greenhouse gas emissions. By choosing more plant-based meals, you're not only taking care of your body but also making a positive impact on the environment. This dual benefit makes plant-based diets an appealing choice for those looking to live more consciously.

Transitioning to a plant-based lifestyle doesn't need to be overwhelming. Start small, and consider initiatives like Meatless Monday. This approach encourages you to dedicate just one day a week to plant-based meals, easing you into the transition. Over time, you might find yourself exploring new flavors and ingredients, broadening your culinary horizons. Another practical tip is to substitute plant proteins for meat in your favorite dishes. Think about replacing ground beef with lentils in your spaghetti sauce or using chickpeas in your salads instead of chicken. These swaps are simple yet effective, allowing you to enjoy familiar meals while incorporating more plant-based options. Gradually, these small changes can add up, leading to a more balanced and plant-focused diet.

When adopting a plant-based lifestyle, it's important to focus on key nutrients to ensure you're meeting your body's needs. Protein is often a concern for those new to plant-based diets, but there's a wide array of plant-based protein sources available. Legumes such as lentils, beans, and chickpeas are excellent choices, as are nuts, seeds, and tofu. Quinoa, a complete protein, is another versatile option. Additionally, keep an eye on vitamin B12, a nutrient primarily found in animal products. B12 is crucial for nerve function and red blood cell production, so consider supplementation or fortified foods to maintain adequate levels. By paying attention to these nutrients, you can maintain a balanced and healthy diet while embracing a plant-based lifestyle.

Misconceptions about plant-based nutrition can sometimes deter people from making the switch. One common myth is that plant-based diets are protein-deficient. However, a varied diet that includes a range of plant-based proteins can easily meet your protein needs. It's all about balance and diversity, ensuring that your meals include a mix of legumes, grains, vegetables, and other protein-rich foods. Another misconception is that plant-based eating is bland or restrictive. In reality, it's an opportunity to experiment with new recipes and flavors, transforming simple ingredients into delicious and satisfying meals. By debunking these myths, you can approach plant-based nutrition with confidence and creativity.

Embracing plant-based nutrition is a journey of discovery, both for your palate and your well-being. As you explore the possibilities, you'll find that plant-based eating is not only healthful but also deeply satisfying. It encourages you to engage with your food, experimenting with textures and flavors that might have been previously overlooked. This approach fosters a mindful relationship with eating, aligning with a holistic lifestyle that values self-care and sustainability. Each plant-based meal is a step toward a healthier you and a healthier planet, creating a ripple effect of positive change.

Balancing Ethical Eating with Personal Health

Navigating the intersection of ethical eating and personal health can sometimes feel like a tightrope walk. On one hand, you want to make choices that reflect your values, like reducing your carbon footprint or supporting fair labor practices. On the other hand, your body has nutritional needs that must be met for you to thrive. This balance can seem daunting, especially if you have personal dietary restrictions, such as allergies or intolerances, that further complicate your choices. The key is to prioritize a balanced diet that provides all the nutrients you need while still honoring your ethical commitments. It's about creating a diet that satisfies both your conscience and your body's requirements.

One approach to achieving this balance is embracing a flexitarian lifestyle, which focuses on reducing meat consumption without eliminating it entirely. This diet allows for flexibility, letting you enjoy plant-based meals most of the time while still partaking in your favorite non-plant dishes. By incorporating diverse food sources, like legumes, grains, and vegetables, you can ensure that your diet is rich in essential nutrients. This variety not only meets your nutritional needs but also supports ethical eating by reducing reliance on resource-intensive animal products. The flexitarian approach is particularly suitable for those who want to make a difference without committing to a fully plant-based lifestyle.

Moderation plays a crucial role in maintaining this balance. It's about acknowledging that occasional indulgences are part of life and don't have to derail your ethical eating goals. Allow yourself to enjoy a non-ethical choice now and then, whether it's a special occasion or a craving you can't shake. The key is to keep these indulgences rare and mindful, ensuring they don't become the norm. By practicing moderation, you can enjoy the foods you love without compromising your ethical values or your health. It's a realistic approach that lets you savor life's pleasures while staying grounded in your principles.

Consider the Mediterranean diet, often hailed as a model of balanced and ethical eating. It emphasizes whole foods, like fruits, vegetables, whole grains, and healthy fats, while incorporating sustainably sourced fish and poultry. This diet highlights the importance of quality over quantity, focusing on fresh, local, and seasonal ingredients that support both health and the environment. Similarly, a plant-forward omnivorous diet allows for a flexible approach, prioritizing plant-based meals while occasionally including ethically sourced animal products. These diets serve as examples of how you can enjoy diverse, satisfying meals that align with both ethical and health-conscious goals.

Balancing ethical eating with personal health is a dynamic process, requiring you to adapt and adjust as needed. It encourages you to be mindful of your choices, both for your health and for the planet. By exploring various dietary options and experimenting with new foods, you can find a balance that's uniquely yours. This balance is not about perfection but about progress, making small, meaningful changes that reflect your values and priorities. As you navigate this path, remember that every choice counts and contributes to a healthier you and a more sustainable world.

Reducing Food Waste: Practical Tips

Imagine you're preparing dinner, chopping vibrant vegetables and arranging them on your counter. But before you know it, you realize that the fridge is filled with forgotten leftovers and expired produce. This is a common scenario, and it contributes significantly to food waste, which has profound environmental consequences. When food ends up in a landfill, it decomposes and releases methane—a potent greenhouse gas—into the atmosphere. This process makes food waste a major contributor to climate change. Moreover, the resources used to produce this wasted food—water, energy, and labor—are also squandered. Think about the energy it takes to grow, harvest, transport, and store food that is ultimately discarded. This wastefulness strains our planet's finite resources and emphasizes the need for change.

At home, there are practical strategies you can adopt to minimize food waste. Meal planning is a simple yet effective method. By planning your meals for the week, you can create a shopping list that ensures you only buy what you need. This approach prevents over-purchasing and reduces the likelihood of food going bad before you can use it. Alongside meal planning, proper storage techniques play a vital role in extending the freshness of your food. For instance, storing fruits and vegetables in the right humidity settings in your fridge can significantly prolong their shelf life. Airtight containers for grains and cereals help maintain their quality, keeping them fresh and ready for use.

Leftovers, often seen as a burden, can actually be an opportunity for culinary creativity. Instead of letting them languish in the back of the fridge, consider how they can be transformed into new meals. Last night's roasted chicken, for example, can become today's chicken salad or tomorrow's hearty soup. By thinking creatively, you can turn leftovers into exciting dishes that save both time and money. Composting is another effective strategy for reducing food waste. By composting food scraps, you can divert waste from landfills and create nutrient-rich soil for gardening. This process not only reduces methane emissions but also enriches the soil, supporting a more sustainable ecosystem.

Community initiatives can amplify these efforts, making a significant impact on food waste reduction. Food sharing networks, for instance, connect individuals with surplus food to those in need, ensuring that excess food finds a home instead of a landfill. These networks promote a sense of community and generosity, transforming potential waste into valuable resources. Supporting food recovery programs is another way to contribute. These programs work with local businesses and organizations to redistribute surplus food to charities and food banks. By participating in or supporting these initiatives, you play a part in creating a more sustainable and equitable food system.

Interactive Journal: Food Waste Reduction Challenge

For one week, challenge yourself to reduce food waste at home. Here's how:

1. *Plan your meals and stick to your shopping list.*

2. *Organize your fridge to ensure older items are used first.*

3. *Get creative with leftovers, making them into new meals.*

4. *Start a compost bin for food scraps.*

By actively engaging in these practices, you not only minimize waste but also develop a deeper appreciation for the food you consume. Each small action contributes to a larger movement towards sustainability, proving that individual efforts can lead to collective change.

Reflection on My Eating Experience Next time you prepare a meal, take a moment to reflect on how you typically eat. Do you eat quickly, distracted, or mindlessly? How does that affect your overall satisfaction with the meal?

Mindful Tasting Exercise As you prepare your next meal, plan to engage in a mindful tasting session:

1. **Focus on the First Bite:** Pay attention to the flavors, textures, and aromas of your food.

2. **Savor Each Bite:** Take your time and notice how the food changes as you chew.

3. **Pause Between Bites:** Put your fork down and breathe before taking the next bite.

Observations During Mindful Eating What did you notice about your food when you ate mindfully? Did you feel more connected to the meal? How did the experience differ from your usual eating habits?

Impact on Satisfaction and Awareness How did slowing down and being mindful of your food affect your sense of satisfaction? What new appreciation or awareness did you gain from the experience?

Small Steps to Cultivate Mindful Eating What small adjustments can you make to incorporate mindful tasting into your routine? How can you create a more intentional eating environment moving forward?

Final Thoughts How does it feel to practice mindful tasting? What benefits do you hope to experience by making it a regular habit?

Music Suggestions Pair this mindful eating experience with soothing music for relaxation and focus:

- **For Tranquil Focus:** *Sunset Lover* by Petit Biscuit

- **For Calm and Presence:** *Weightless* by Marconi Union

- **For Light and Uplifting Energy:** *Better Together* by Jack Johnson

Sustainable Sourcing: Making Informed Choices

Imagine standing in your local market, surrounded by an array of vibrant produce. Each item represents more than just food; it embodies a choice that impacts both your health and the planet's future. Sustainable sourcing is about those choices. It involves obtaining ingredients in a way that maintains the long-term viability of food systems and preserves biodiversity. This approach ensures that the land, waters, and ecosystems used in food production remain healthy for future generations. By prioritizing sustainability, we can support practices that protect natural resources and promote ecological balance. This way, the food we enjoy today doesn't compromise the ability of future generations to enjoy the same.

Identifying sustainably sourced products can feel daunting, but there are tools to guide you. Eco-labels and certifications provide insight into the practices behind your food. Certifications like Rainforest Alliance and Marine Stewardship Council ensure that products are produced with minimal environmental impact, promoting ethical and sustainable farming methods. Transparency and accountability are crucial, too. Brands that openly share their sourcing practices and maintain traceable supply chains offer reassurance about the sustainability of their products. By seeking out these labels and supporting brands that prioritize sustainability, you can make informed choices that align with your values and contribute to a healthier planet.

Consumer demand plays a pivotal role in promoting sustainability. As consumers, we have the power to drive market change through our purchasing decisions. When we support brands that embrace sustainable practices, we send a clear message about the importance of environmental responsibility. This demand encourages more companies to adopt sustainable sourcing, creating a ripple effect that can transform entire industries. Whether it's choosing a company that prioritizes ethical labor practices or one that focuses on reducing carbon emissions, your choices matter. They can inspire widespread adoption of sustainable practices, benefiting both the environment and the communities involved in food production.

Consider the success stories of sustainable sourcing practices that have made a significant impact. Community-supported agriculture programs connect consumers directly with local farmers, providing access to fresh, seasonal produce while supporting small-scale, sustainable farming. These programs reduce the distance food travels, minimizing its carbon footprint and fostering local economic growth. Another example is sustainable seafood sourcing, which focuses on harvesting fish in ways that maintain healthy populations and ecosystems. Initiatives like these demonstrate how sustainable sourcing can create positive change, benefiting both the environment and those who rely on it for their livelihoods. By participating in such programs, you contribute to a movement that supports sustainability and promotes responsible stewardship of natural resources.

The Environmental Impact of Dietary Choices

When you think about what you eat, it's easy to focus just on taste and nutrition. But your meal choices also play a crucial role in shaping the environment. Different diets come with varying ecological footprints. For instance, plant-based diets typically have a smaller environmental impact compared to meat-heavy diets. This is largely because producing meat, especially beef, involves significant resources like water and land, resulting in high greenhouse gas emissions.

In contrast, plant-based foods require fewer resources and produce less pollution, making them a more sustainable choice. Yet, it's not just about meat vs. plants. Monoculture crops, such as corn and soy, often used to feed livestock, can also harm the environment. They contribute to soil degradation and biodiversity loss, creating a complex web of environmental challenges tied to our food choices. Understanding these impacts helps you make informed decisions, not just for your health, but for the planet.

There are practical strategies you can adopt to reduce the environmental impact of your diet. One effective approach is to prioritize local and seasonal foods. These options are often fresher and require less energy for transportation and storage. By choosing what's in season, you also support local farmers and reduce the carbon footprint of your meals. Additionally, cutting back on processed foods is beneficial. Processing often involves extra energy and resources, not to mention packaging that can end up in landfills. Instead, focus on whole foods that are closer to their natural state. They not only have a lower environmental impact but also offer better nutrition. Making these simple changes can have a significant positive effect on the environment.

Considering the carbon-conscious aspect of your diet can further guide your choices. A carbon-conscious diet focuses on reducing the carbon footprint of your meals. You can start by calculating the carbon impact of the foods you eat. There are various online tools and resources that can help you understand which foods have higher carbon emissions and why. Once you have this knowledge, you can plan low-carbon meals, emphasizing foods with lower emissions. This might mean more plant-based dishes or incorporating sustainably sourced fish and poultry. It's about making thoughtful choices that align with sustainability goals. By being mindful of the carbon footprint of your diet, you contribute to a healthier planet.

To put these ideas into practice, consider engaging in environmentally conscious dietary habits. Participating in community gardens is a great way to access fresh, local produce while reducing reliance on commercially grown foods. These gardens foster community spirit and offer opportunities to learn about sustainable agriculture. Another impactful practice is supporting regenerative agriculture. This method focuses on regenerating soil health and enhancing ecosystem biodiversity. By choosing products from farms that use regenerative practices, you support a system that prioritizes long-term environmental health. These practices remind us that our food choices extend beyond our plates, influencing the world around us in profound ways.

As we wrap up this chapter, it's clear that our dietary choices are deeply intertwined with environmental health. From reducing carbon footprints to supporting sustainable farming, what we eat matters not just for our bodies but for the planet. Embracing eco-friendly habits is part of a broader commitment to wellness, one that considers both personal health and global impact. With these insights, you're equipped to make choices that reflect a holistic approach to well-being, leading seamlessly into our next chapter on interactive journaling for self-discovery.

Chapter 7

Interactive Journaling for Self-Discovery

Imagine for a moment that you're in a bustling café, a steaming cup of coffee beside you, and a journal open in front of you. It's not just a blank page; it's a canvas for your thoughts, a place where your inner world meets the outer one. Journaling is more than just jotting down events of the day. It's a tool for understanding yourself, a way to sift through the noise and distill your experiences into something meaningful. In our fast-paced lives, where everything demands our attention, taking a moment to write can feel like a breath of fresh air, a pause that allows you to reflect and recalibrate.

Reflective journaling is a process where you pour your thoughts and emotions onto paper, clarifying them in the process. It acts as a mirror, allowing you to see your thoughts more clearly and develop a deeper understanding of your feelings. By consistently journaling, you enhance your self-awareness, recognizing patterns and triggers in your behavior that might otherwise go unnoticed. This practice encourages introspection, helping you make sense of complex emotions and experiences. In doing so, you gain insight into yourself, fostering a greater sense of self-acceptance and understanding.

The mental health benefits of journaling are well-documented. Regular journaling can reduce stress and anxiety by providing a safe outlet for expressing emotions. When you write about your fears, worries, or frustrations, you externalize them, reducing their power over you. This act of expression can lead to improved mood and emotional regulation, helping you navigate life's challenges with more resilience. Studies have shown that expressive writing can lower blood pressure, improve lung and liver function, and even reduce depressive symptoms. By incorporating journaling into your routine, you create a space for emotional release and healing, promoting overall well-being and mental clarity.

Supporting the benefits of journaling, research has demonstrated its therapeutic potency. Engaging in expressive writing can significantly reduce depressive symptoms, enhance mood, and contribute to better overall physical health. This approach, free from medication, is increasingly being incorporated into psychotherapy to assist in the management of anxiety, depression, and stress. Journaling fosters a welcoming space for mental experiences, aiding in psychological well-being and therapeutic success. The act of recording one's thoughts and emotions initiates a journey of introspection and growth, leading to a healthier mind and a more understood self. The advantages of keeping a journal go far beyond providing temporary solace, opening doors to lasting self-discovery and deeper comprehension.

There are various styles of journaling you can explore, each offering its own unique benefits. Free-writing, for instance, is a stream-of-consciousness approach where you let your thoughts flow without worrying about structure or grammar. This method allows you to tap into your subconscious, uncovering insights that might be hidden beneath the surface. It's about unfiltered expression, capturing the essence of your thoughts and emotions as they arise. On the other hand, structured journaling involves using prompts to guide your writing. These prompts can help focus your reflections, encouraging you to delve into specific themes or aspects of your life. By providing a framework, structured journaling allows you to explore your thoughts more deeply, fostering greater clarity and understanding.

Interactive Exercise: Journaling Starter Prompts

Set aside 10 minutes each day to explore your thoughts through journaling. Start with these prompts: "What is one thing I learned about myself today?" and "What emotions did I experi-

ence, and why?" Try both free-writing and structured approaches to discover what resonates with you. This practice is not about perfection; it's about creating a dialogue with yourself, a conversation that unfolds on the page. As you engage with these prompts, allow yourself to be curious and open, letting your insights guide you toward greater self-awareness and personal growth.

Reflection on My Nutrition Tracking Take a moment to reflect on your current approach to nutrition. Do you find yourself guessing what's in your meals, or do you have a system in place? How do you track your food, if at all? How accurate or helpful do you find your current method?

What's Working Well Write down what you think works well in your current nutrition tracking. Are there any habits or tools that help you make healthier food choices?

Areas to Improve Reflect on areas where you feel your tracking could improve. Do you miss meals or forget to log certain items? Are there any gaps that leave you unsure about your nutrient intake?

The Role of Digital Tools Consider how a digital tool could support your goals. Would it help with meal planning, nutrient tracking, or accountability? How might an app streamline your process and make tracking easier?

Choosing the Right App Identify any needs or features that you would like a nutrition app to have. Would you prefer one with barcode scanning, meal suggestions, or nutrient breakdowns?

Small Steps to Improve Tracking What small steps can you take today to improve your nutrition tracking? Could you try a new app or make a habit of tracking after each meal?

Final Thoughts How does tracking your nutrition make you feel? What do you hope to achieve with a more structured approach to tracking your meals?

Music Suggestions Pair this reflection with soothing or motivational music for focus:

- *For Focus and Calm*: *Weightless* by Marconi Union

- *For Motivation and Clarity*: *Good Life* by OneRepublic

- *For Relaxation*: *Sunset Lover* by Petit Biscuit

This journaling practice allows you to slow down, reflect, and gain insights that support your personal growth and mindfulness journey.

Journaling Prompts for Mindful Eating

Picture yourself at the dinner table, plate full of vibrant colors, each bite a sensory delight. Yet, how often do we really tune into the experience of eating? Journaling can transform this everyday act into a mindful practice, helping you become more aware of your eating habits and patterns. It's not just about what you eat, but how and why. By journaling, you can uncover emotional triggers that prompt you to reach for food, whether it's stress, boredom, or even joy. This awareness is crucial, as it allows you to reflect on your eating experiences, helping you distinguish between physical hunger and emotional cravings. Writing about these moments can reveal patterns you might not have noticed, fostering a healthier relationship with food.

To guide you on this path, consider using specific prompts to explore your relationship with eating. Start by asking, "What emotions do I feel before, during, and after eating?" This question encourages you to pause and assess your emotional state, offering insights into your motivations for eating. Another powerful prompt is, "How does my body feel after each meal?" Reflecting on your body's physical responses can help you understand the effects of different foods, promoting better choices in the future. These prompts serve as gentle guides, leading you to deeper insights into your eating habits. They encourage you to slow down and engage with your meals, turning eating into a mindful practice rather than a hurried task.

Using prompts can be incredibly beneficial, offering a structured way to engage with your thoughts and feelings around food. They act as anchors, focusing your reflections and helping you uncover the "why" behind your eating habits. This practice can lead to mindful eating, where you savor each bite and listen to your body's hunger cues. By regularly engaging with these prompts, you develop a habit of mindfulness that extends beyond mealtimes, influencing your approach to food and health. The insights gained through journaling can empower you to make conscious choices, fostering a balanced and intuitive way of eating.

Integrating journaling into your mealtime routine doesn't have to be complicated. Consider starting with a pre-meal reflection exercise. Before you begin eating, take a moment to jot down your hunger level and emotional state. Are you truly hungry, or are you eating for another reason? This simple practice can ground you in the present moment, aligning your eating with your body's needs. After your meal, engage in a post-meal journaling session. Reflect on how the meal made you feel, both physically and emotionally. Did it satisfy your hunger? Did it bring you joy or comfort? By dedicating a few minutes to these reflections, you create a mindful space that enhances your connection to food.

Transforming your eating habits through journaling is a journey of self-discovery. It's about cultivating a deeper understanding of what drives your food choices and how they affect your well-being. By incorporating these practices into your daily routine, you foster a sense of mindfulness that extends to all areas of your life. Each meal becomes an opportunity to explore and learn, guiding you toward a more intuitive and balanced approach to eating. As you continue to engage with these prompts, you'll find that they not only enhance your relationship with food but also support your overall health and happiness.

Tracking Emotional Well-Being

Picture your emotions as waves, constantly shifting and changing, sometimes calm and sometimes tumultuous. Keeping track of these emotional tides through an emotional well-being journal can be a powerful tool for understanding your mental health. By doing so, you gain insights into your patterns and mood fluctuations, recognizing what triggers certain emotional responses. This awareness becomes invaluable, allowing you to anticipate how you might feel in different scenarios and prepare accordingly. Think of it as a map that charts your emotional landscape, guiding you through the peaks and valleys that we all experience in life.

To effectively track your emotional states, consider incorporating daily mood charts into your routine. These visual tools allow you to record your feelings on a scale—maybe from one to ten—giving you a clear picture of how your emotions ebb and flow over time. Another useful technique is the emotion wheel, a colorful chart that helps identify and expand on basic feelings like happiness, anger, or sadness, encouraging you to explore the nuances of your emotions. By labeling your feelings more precisely, you begin to understand the complexity of your emotional experiences, which can lead to greater clarity and acceptance of your mental states.

Understanding emotional patterns through tracking can significantly enhance your well-being. As you become more attuned to your emotional rhythms, you learn to anticipate and manage your responses more effectively. This anticipation allows you to prepare for challenging situations, equipping you with strategies to cope when emotions run high. Moreover, tracking emotions increases your emotional intelligence, helping you recognize not just your feelings but also the emotions of those around you. This awareness can improve your relationships, as you become more empathetic and understanding in your interactions with others.

To support your emotional journaling practice, explore various tools and resources that cater to different preferences and lifestyles. Mood tracking apps, for instance, are convenient options for those who prefer digital solutions. Apps like MoodPath or Daylio offer features that allow you to log your emotions throughout the day, often including prompts or questions to guide your reflections. For those who enjoy a more tactile approach, bullet journaling templates for emotions provide a structured yet customizable layout for recording your feelings. These templates can be tailored to your needs, offering a creative outlet that encourages regular engagement with your emotional tracking practice.

Consider incorporating an interactive element, such as a checklist to help establish your emotional tracking routine. Begin by selecting a method that resonates with you, whether it's a digital app or a paper journal. Commit to logging your emotions at least once a day, perhaps at a consistent time like morning or evening. Use your mood tracker to note any patterns, triggers, or significant events that influence your emotional state. Over time, reflect on the data you've gathered to identify recurring themes or insights. This checklist serves as a guide to ensure that your emotional tracking becomes a habit, supporting your journey toward greater self-awareness and emotional balance.

Visualizing Your Health Goals

Picture yourself standing on a mountaintop, the wind in your hair, and a clear vision of where you want to be in your wellness journey. Visualization is a powerful tool that can transform your goals from distant dreams into tangible realities. By clearly imagining your desired outcomes, you create a mental blueprint that guides your actions and decisions. This process isn't just about daydreaming—it's about harnessing the mind's ability to influence your motivation and clarity. Visualization connects your intentions with your achievements, making your goals feel more attainable and less abstract. When you visualize success, you're not just hoping for it; you're actively preparing your mind to recognize opportunities and overcome obstacles. This practice instills a sense of confidence, reinforcing your commitment to your health goals and helping you stay focused on what truly matters.

To bring your visions to life, consider using techniques that create a vivid mental picture of your desired outcomes. Vision boards are a popular method, where you gather images and words that represent your health and wellness aspirations. These boards serve as a visual reminder, keeping your goals at the forefront of your mind. Whether it's a picture of a serene yoga pose or a quote about resilience, each element on your board should resonate with your personal journey. Guided visualization exercises are another effective approach, where you close your eyes and immerse yourself in a detailed mental scenario of achieving your goals. Imagine the sights, sounds, and emotions associated with reaching your desired state of health. By engaging your senses, you make the experience more real, enhancing your motivation to work towards it.

The benefits of goal visualization are profound, as this practice can significantly reinforce your commitment and focus. When you regularly visualize your goals, you create a mental rehearsal that prepares you for success. This rehearsal boosts your confidence, as your mind becomes accustomed to the idea of achieving what you set out to do. The vivid imagery associated with visualization can reignite your motivation during times of doubt or challenge. It reminds you of the reasons behind your efforts, helping you push through obstacles with renewed determination. Visualization transforms your aspirations from mere wishes into actionable plans, solidifying your resolve to pursue them with dedication and passion.

To make visualization a regular part of your routine, incorporate practical exercises that align with your goals. Creating a collage of health aspirations is a creative way to engage with your vision. Gather magazines, printouts, or even your own drawings that symbolize your wellness dreams, and arrange them on a board or in a journal. This tactile activity encourages reflection and reinforces your goals each time you see it. Another exercise involves daily affirmation practices related to your goals. Start each day with positive statements that affirm your commitment to your health journey. Whether spoken aloud or written down, these affirmations serve as a reminder of your intentions and encourage a mindset of positivity and possibility.

Visualization is more than a practice—it's a mindset that empowers you to take charge of your health and well-being. By vividly picturing your goals, you create a mental landscape where success feels not only possible but inevitable. This mindset fosters resilience, motivating you to navigate challenges with grace and determination. As you continue to engage with visualization, you'll find that it enhances your ability to stay focused, inspired, and aligned with your aspirations. Each visualization session strengthens your belief in yourself and your capacity to achieve the outcomes you desire. With this powerful tool at your disposal, you're equipped to transform your health goals into a fulfilling reality.

Gratitude Practices for Positivity

Imagine waking up and, instead of diving headfirst into the day's to-do list, you take a moment to acknowledge what you're grateful for. This small shift in focus can transform your entire outlook. Gratitude is a powerful tool that can help shift your attention from what's lacking in life to the abundance you already have. By practicing gratitude, you develop a positive mindset that reduces negative thinking patterns. It's like training your brain to see the glass as half full, focusing on the silver linings rather than the clouds. Gratitude encourages you to pause and appreciate the good, even amidst stress or uncertainty. This shift in perspective can lead to a more optimistic and contented life.

One effective way to cultivate gratitude is through regular journaling exercises. Start by writing down three things you're grateful for each day. These don't have to be grand gestures; they can be as simple as a warm cup of coffee, a smile from a stranger, or a moment of peace in your hectic schedule. By recording these moments, you create a tangible record of positivity that you can revisit whenever you need a boost. Reflecting on positive interactions with others is another powerful exercise. Think about a recent conversation that uplifted you or an act of kindness you received. Write about how it made you feel and why it mattered to you. These reflections not only enhance your appreciation for the present but also strengthen your connections with those around you.

The benefits of gratitude extend far beyond the journal page. Practicing gratitude can enhance emotional resilience, helping you bounce back from setbacks with greater ease.

When you focus on the positive, you cultivate a mindset of abundance, which can improve your relational well-being. You become more empathetic and understanding, as gratitude encourages you to see the good in people and situations. This shift in perspective can lead to stronger, more fulfilling relationships, as you approach interactions with kindness and appreciation. Gratitude also fosters a sense of contentment, reducing the tendency to compare yourself to others and increasing satisfaction with your own life.

Integrating gratitude into your daily life doesn't have to be a daunting task. Consider starting a gratitude journal that you write in before bed. This simple practice allows you to end the day on a positive note, reflecting on the good things that happened and setting the stage for a restful night's sleep. Sharing gratitude with friends or family is another wonderful way to make it a habit. Perhaps over dinner, you each share one thing you're thankful for, turning gratitude into a shared experience. This practice not only strengthens your relationships but also creates a supportive environment where positivity is celebrated and encouraged.

As you incorporate these gratitude practices into your routine, you'll likely notice a shift in how you perceive and interact with the world. The more you focus on the positive aspects of life, the more they'll multiply, creating a cycle of joy and appreciation. Gratitude becomes a lens through which you view your experiences, transforming challenges into opportunities for growth and connection. This practice is not about ignoring difficulties but rather about finding the good amidst the chaos. By embracing gratitude, you open yourself up to a world of positivity and possibility, enriching your life in ways you may not have imagined.

Creating a Personalized Wellness Journal

Imagine your wellness journal as a trusted companion on your path to health. It's not just a collection of pages; it's a personalized space that reflects your unique journey, goals, and values. By customizing your journal, you create a tailored guide that aligns with your aspirations and needs. This personalization is key, as it ensures that every entry, every thought, and every plan resonates with who you are and what you aim to achieve. Your journal becomes a reflection of your personal wellness narrative, capturing the essence of your journey toward holistic health.

Setting up your wellness journal involves thoughtful design and organization, turning it into a tool that supports your growth. Start by selecting sections for different aspects of wellness that matter to you, such as nutrition, exercise, mental health, and personal growth. Each section offers a dedicated space to explore and document your progress, creating a comprehensive overview of your wellness journey. Incorporate inspirational quotes or images that resonate with your goals, infusing your journal with motivation and positivity. These visual elements serve as daily reminders of your aspirations, encouraging you to stay focused and inspired. By organizing your journal in this way, you create a tool that not only supports your wellness goals but also inspires and uplifts you along the way.

The power of a personalized journal lies in its ability to enhance motivation and engagement, offering a sense of ownership and accountability. When your journal aligns with your personal wellness goals, it becomes a source of inspiration, guiding you toward meaningful change. The customization process encourages you to take ownership of your journey, fostering a deeper connection with your goals. This alignment increases accountability, as the journal becomes a tangible representation of your commitment to health and well-being. By regularly engaging with your personalized journal, you maintain momentum and focus, propelling you forward on your path to holistic health.

Consider exploring creative journal layouts that make your wellness journey engaging and functional. Monthly goal-setting pages can help you outline your aspirations and track your progress, providing a clear roadmap for your wellness journey. These pages offer a space to set intentions, reflect on achievements, and adjust your goals as needed. Wellness trackers for habits and progress are another valuable addition, allowing you to monitor behaviors and celebrate milestones. These trackers provide visual feedback on your efforts, reinforcing positive habits and motivating you to continue. By incorporating these elements into your journal, you create a dynamic and interactive tool that supports your wellness journey in a meaningful way.

As you continue to engage with your personalized wellness journal, you'll discover its capacity to transform your approach to health and well-being. The journal becomes a living document that evolves with you, capturing your growth and achievements. It serves as a reminder of your resilience, adaptability, and dedication to personal growth. This journey of self-discovery and wellness is not just about reaching a destination; it's about embracing the process and finding joy in each step. A personalized journal is more than a record of your journey; it's a celebration of your commitment to living a balanced and fulfilling life.

Your personalized wellness journal is a powerful tool that supports your journey toward holistic health. By customizing its design and incorporating elements that resonate with you, you create a journal that reflects your unique path. This personalization enhances motivation and engagement, aligning the journal with your wellness goals and fostering accountability. As you explore creative layouts and track your progress, you'll find that your journal becomes an invaluable companion on your journey to health and well-being. It captures your growth, celebrates your achievements, and inspires you to continue moving forward with confidence and determination.

Chapter 8

Enhancing Your Wellness Journey with Technology

Think back to the last time you felt the rush of excitement when starting something new—a new project, hobby, or perhaps a fitness routine. That initial burst of motivation can be invigorating, but as days turn into weeks, maintaining that momentum often becomes the real challenge. This is where technology can be your steadfast ally, bridging the gap between initial enthusiasm and long-term commitment. In today's fast-paced world, where schedules are packed to the brim, fitness apps offer a convenient and engaging solution to keep you accountable and motivated. These digital tools provide reminders, track progress, and even sprinkle in a bit of fun to keep you on track.

Fitness apps have become invaluable for those of us seeking to stay committed to our health goals amidst life's chaos.

They act as a personal coach tucked right in your pocket, guiding you with reminders and tracking your every step or calorie. Imagine having a virtual cheerleader that not only nudges you to get moving but also celebrates your accomplishments, big or small. Many apps seamlessly integrate with wearable devices, enhancing their effectiveness by providing real-time feedback on your activity levels. This integration allows you to set personalized goals and receive instant notifications, making it easier to stay informed and motivated. Whether you're running a marathon or simply aiming to increase your daily step count, these apps are designed to help you stay the course.

The concept of gamification in fitness apps takes motivation to another level. By introducing elements like reward systems and achievement badges, these apps make fitness feel less like a chore and more like a game. Imagine completing a workout and earning a badge that signifies your progress, or participating in virtual challenges that push you to achieve new milestones. These gamified elements tap into our innate desire to achieve and excel, transforming workouts into engaging and rewarding activities. Virtual competitions add an extra layer of excitement, allowing you to challenge friends or join global events, creating a sense of accountability and friendly rivalry that keeps you coming back for more.

When selecting the right fitness app, it's important to consider your personal goals and preferences. Start by evaluating the features each app offers—look for those that align with your fitness objectives and lifestyle. User reviews can provide valuable insights into the app's usability and effectiveness, helping you make an informed decision. It's also wise to try free versions of apps before committing to a paid subscription. This allows you to explore the interface, test the features, and determine whether the app truly meets your needs. Remember, the best app is one that seamlessly integrates into your daily routine, offering support and motivation without adding unnecessary complexity.

Interactive Journal: Fitness App Evaluation Checklist

- *Identify Your Goals: Determine your primary fitness objectives, such as weight loss, muscle gain, or increased endurance.*

- *Research Features: Look for apps with features that support your goals, such as workout plans, progress tracking, or social elements.*

- *Read User Reviews: Gain insights from other users regarding the app's effectiveness and usability.*

- *Test Free Versions: Try free versions or trial periods to evaluate the app's interface and features.*

- *Consider Integration: Ensure the app can sync with your wearable devices for enhanced tracking and engagement.*

- *Assess Community Aspects: Decide if social connectivity and community challenges are important to you in maintaining motivation.*

Digital Tools for Tracking Nutrition

Imagine standing in front of your pantry, trying to decide what to have for dinner. You want something nutritious, but after a long day, the last thing you want is to spend more time than necessary thinking about food. This is where digital tools for nutrition tracking come into play, simplifying the process of monitoring your dietary habits. With just a few taps on your smartphone, you can log your meals, scan barcodes for instant nutritional information, and even track your macro and micronutrient intake. These tools take the guesswork out of eating, allowing you to focus on enjoying your meals instead of worrying about them. Whether you're aiming to lose weight, maintain your current health, or reach new nutritional goals, these apps can provide the structure you need to stay on track.

Among the myriad of apps available, some stand out for their specific offerings. Lose It! is perfect for weight management, providing a straightforward platform to set goals and monitor your progress. It's user-friendly, with a database that helps you log foods quickly. If you're someone who needs detailed nutrient analysis, Cronometer is an excellent choice. It breaks down both macro and micronutrients, offering insights into your diet's nutritional profile and highlighting any deficiencies. For those who like to plan ahead, Yazio can be a game-changer. It not only helps you track what you eat but also assists in meal planning, catering to specific diets or preferences. By utilizing these apps, you gain access to a wealth of information that can help you make informed dietary choices tailored to your lifestyle and health needs.

Integrating nutrition data with your fitness goals can give you a comprehensive view of your health, allowing you to see how what you eat affects your physical performance. Many nutrition apps sync with fitness trackers, providing an all-encompassing picture of your daily activity and nutrition. By analyzing this data, you can adjust your dietary plans to better support your workouts, ensuring you're fueling your body appropriately. This integration fosters a deeper understanding of how your lifestyle choices interconnect, helping you make adjustments that lead to more balanced, effective health practices. When you see how your nutrition impacts your energy levels and workout recovery, you can tailor your meals to optimize performance and well-being.

Maintaining consistency in tracking can be a challenge, but with a few strategies, it becomes a sustainable habit. Setting daily reminders on your phone can prompt you to log meals and snacks consistently, making it part of your routine. Pre-logging meals can also help, especially if you have a regular eating schedule. By planning your meals ahead of time, you reduce the temptation to stray from your nutritional goals and ensure that you're prepared with healthy options. This approach not only keeps you accountable but also simplifies decision-making, reducing the stress associated with meal planning. The key is to find a rhythm that works for you, one that fits seamlessly into your daily life without feeling like a chore.

Interactive Element: Nutrition Tracking Reflection Prompt

Take a moment to reflect on your current approach to nutrition. Do you find yourself guessing what's in your meals, or do you have a system in place? Write down what you think works well and areas you'd like to improve. Then, consider how a digital tool could support your goals. Would it help with meal planning, nutrient tracking, or accountability? Identifying your needs can guide you to the right app, enhancing your nutritional habits with ease and precision.

Reflection on My Nutrition Tracking Take a moment to reflect on your current approach to nutrition. Do you find yourself guessing what's in your meals, or do you have a system in place? How do you track your food, if at all? How accurate or helpful do you find your current method?

What's Working Well Write down what you think works well in your current nutrition tracking. Are there any habits or tools that help you make healthier food choices?

Areas to Improve Reflect on areas where you feel your tracking could improve. Do you miss meals or forget to log certain items? Are there any gaps that leave you unsure about your nutrient intake?

The Role of Digital Tools Consider how a digital tool could support your goals. Would it help with meal planning, nutrient tracking, or accountability? How might an app streamline your process and make tracking easier?

Choosing the Right App Identify any needs or features that you would like a nutrition app to have. Would you prefer one with barcode scanning, meal suggestions, or nutrient breakdowns?

Small Steps to Improve Tracking What small steps can you take today to improve your nutrition tracking? Could you try a new app or make a habit of tracking after each meal?

Final Thoughts How does tracking your nutrition make you feel? What do you hope to achieve with a more structured approach to tracking your meals?

Music Suggestions Pair this reflection with soothing or motivational music for focus:

- *For Focus and Calm*: *Weightless* by Marconi Union
- *For Motivation and Clarity*: *Good Life* by OneRepublic
- *For Relaxation*: *Sunset Lover* by Petit Biscuit

Online Communities for Support and Motivation

Picture this: you've just completed a grueling workout, and while you feel accomplished, a part of you wishes you could share the moment with someone who truly gets it. Enter online communities—digital spaces that connect like-minded individuals who share your passion for wellness. These communities are more than just forums; they're hubs of support and motivation. They offer a unique blend of camaraderie and accountability, making your wellness journey less solitary and more social. Whether you're swapping workout tips, sharing personal victories, or seeking advice on overcoming challenges, these platforms cultivate a sense of belonging and encouragement.

One of the most vibrant online wellness communities is Reddit's fitness groups. It's a treasure trove of workout tips, advice, and personal stories that resonate with people from all walks of life. Whether you're a seasoned athlete or a fitness newbie, you'll find a wealth of information and inspiration here. App forums are another excellent resource, offering diet support and a chance to connect with others on similar health journeys. These forums are filled with individuals who understand the ups and downs of maintaining a healthy lifestyle, providing a safe space to share experiences and gain insights. Facebook groups focused on specific health goals also play a significant role in fostering supportive environments. From weight loss challenges to plant-based eating, there's a group for every interest, making it easy to find your tribe and stay motivated.

The power of peer support in achieving wellness goals cannot be overstated. Engaging with a community of like-minded individuals enhances accountability and persistence. When you witness others celebrating their successes, it fuels your motivation to keep pushing forward. Collaborative goal-setting becomes a shared endeavor, turning personal milestones into collective achievements. It's not just about ticking off a goal on your list; it's about doing it with the support and encouragement of others who want to see you succeed. This sense of community fosters resilience and commitment, making it easier to stay on track even when the going gets tough.

Finding the right online community can be a game-changer, but it's essential to choose one that aligns with your personal needs and values. Start by assessing the group's dynamics and culture. Are the interactions positive and supportive? Is there a sense of camaraderie and mutual respect? These factors are crucial in ensuring that the community will be a source of encouragement rather than stress. Explore multiple platforms to find the best fit for your goals and personality. Some people thrive in large, bustling forums, while others prefer smaller, more intimate spaces. Take the time to explore different options, and don't be afraid to leave a group if it doesn't feel right. The beauty of online communities lies in their diversity, offering countless opportunities to connect with people who share your passions and aspirations.

Remember, the value of these communities extends beyond immediate support. They provide a platform for lifelong learning and growth, where you can continually expand your knowledge and refine your approach to wellness.

Engaging with others introduces you to new perspectives and ideas, enriching your understanding of health and fitness. Whether it's discovering a new workout routine, learning about a different dietary approach, or simply finding inspiration in someone else's story, these interactions are invaluable. As you navigate your wellness journey, online communities can serve as a constant source of motivation and encouragement, reminding you that you're never alone in your pursuit of health and happiness.

Virtual Workouts: Finding What Works for You

Picture yourself at home, the day winding down, and you realize you haven't had the chance to exercise yet. Instead of feeling guilty for missing a gym session, you remember that you have an entire fitness studio at your fingertips. Virtual workouts have revolutionized how we approach exercise, offering a flexibility that fits seamlessly into our busy lives. They provide the convenience of at-home exercise, eliminating the need for travel and allowing you to work out on your schedule. With just a few clicks, you can access a diverse range of workout styles, from high-intensity interval training to calming yoga sessions, all from the comfort of your living room.

Platforms like Peloton have taken the fitness world by storm, known for their dynamic cycling and cardio classes that make you feel like you're part of a live studio session. The energy of the instructors and the community vibe can turn a regular workout into an exhilarating experience. If variety is what you crave, Beachbody On Demand offers an array of programs, ranging from intense strength training to dance-inspired routines, ensuring there's something for every mood and fitness level. For those seeking a more mindful approach, YogaGlo provides a sanctuary for yoga and meditation, helping you center your mind and body amidst life's chaos. These platforms cater to various preferences, making it easy to find workouts that resonate with your personal interests and fitness goals.

Exploring different workout styles not only keeps things fresh but also helps you discover what truly motivates you. Maybe you've always been a runner, but trying a dance cardio class brings a new level of joy to your routine. Or perhaps strength training has been your go-to, but incorporating some yoga helps balance your body and mind. Experimenting with various formats can reveal new passions and keep your fitness routine from becoming monotonous. It also allows you to adapt your workouts to changing goals. Whether you're training for a specific event, recovering from an injury, or simply seeking variety, the world of virtual workouts offers endless possibilities to tailor your exercise regimen.

Creating an effective virtual workout routine requires a bit of planning but can lead to a balanced and fulfilling fitness practice. Start by combining different types of workouts—strength, cardio, and flexibility—to ensure a well-rounded approach. This mix not only benefits your overall fitness but also keeps your body challenged and engaged. Setting regular workout times is crucial, as it establishes a routine that becomes a natural part of your day. Whether it's a morning session to kickstart your energy or an evening class to unwind, consistency is key. It's about finding a rhythm that suits your lifestyle, making exercise a habit rather than a chore.

To make the most of your virtual workouts, consider the environment where you'll exercise. Create a space that inspires movement, free from distractions and clutter. A simple mat, some weights, or resistance bands can transform any area into a mini gym. The goal is to cultivate a setting where you feel motivated and at ease, enhancing your focus and enjoyment of each session. As you explore the world of virtual workouts, remember that the journey is deeply personal. It's about discovering what moves you, both physically and emotionally, and embracing the freedom and flexibility that technology provides.

Mindfulness Apps to Enhance Meditation

Imagine starting your day with a few moments of quiet reflection, a time to set intentions and center yourself before the hustle and bustle begins. But finding the discipline to meditate consistently can be a challenge, especially when life feels like a whirlwind. Enter mindfulness apps, designed to help you establish and maintain a meditation routine that fits seamlessly into your daily life. These apps offer guided sessions perfect for beginners, taking the guesswork out of meditation and providing a gentle introduction to the practice. With the tap of a finger, you can access a library of meditations tailored to various needs and preferences, allowing you to explore different techniques and find what resonates most with you. Timer functions also cater to those who prefer self-paced practice, offering flexibility and autonomy in your meditation journey.

Among the array of apps available, some have gained popularity for their diverse meditation resources. Headspace is renowned for its structured learning approach, guiding users through meditation basics with ease and clarity. It's a great starting point for those new to mindfulness, offering step-by-step courses that build confidence and understanding. Calm, on the other hand, focuses on providing relaxation and sleep support, making it ideal for winding down after a long day. Its serene soundscapes and bedtime stories create a peaceful environment conducive to relaxation and rest. Insight Timer stands out with its extensive collection of meditations, catering to a wide range of styles and lengths. Whether you have a few minutes or an hour, Insight Timer offers something to suit your schedule and mood. Each app brings its unique strengths, allowing you to tailor your meditation experience to your personal needs and lifestyle.

Beyond the basics, mindfulness apps include features that enrich and deepen your meditation practice. Ambient sounds and music can transform your space into a tranquil retreat, enhancing the meditative experience and helping you focus. Many apps also offer progress tracking and milestones, allowing you to see your growth and stay motivated. As you reach milestones, such as consecutive days of meditation, you gain a sense of accomplishment and encouragement to continue. This progress tracking is more than just a record; it's a visual reminder of your commitment to self-care and inner peace. These features help maintain interest and engagement, making meditation a rewarding and evolving practice.

Incorporating meditation apps into your daily routine doesn't have to be complicated. Consider starting with a morning or evening ritual, dedicating a few minutes to mindfulness before the day begins or as it winds down. This routine can set a positive tone for your day or help you release the stress of daily life. If you find yourself overwhelmed during work, using an app for quick meditation breaks can provide relief and clarity, allowing you to return to tasks with renewed focus and calm. Integrate these moments of mindfulness into your schedule, treating them as essential as any other appointment or commitment. The key is consistency, finding a rhythm that complements your lifestyle and priorities.

Mindfulness apps serve as a bridge between intention and practice, offering tools and guidance to support your meditation journey. They provide a structure that makes meditation accessible to all, regardless of experience level. By incorporating these apps into your routine, you open the door to a world of mindfulness that can transform how you navigate life's challenges and joys. Whether you're seeking relaxation, focus, or personal growth, mindfulness apps offer a wealth of resources to accompany you on your path to self-discovery and tranquility.

Balancing Screen Time with Mindful Living

In today's digital age, screens have become an integral part of our lives, from smartphones and tablets to computers and televisions. While technology brings countless conveniences, it also presents challenges, especially when it comes to mental health. Excessive screen time can lead to digital fatigue, a condition characterized by symptoms such as eye strain, headaches, and mental exhaustion. It's easy to fall into the cycle of endless scrolling or binge-watching, only to find yourself feeling more drained than relaxed. Recognizing these symptoms is crucial for maintaining a healthy balance between technology use and mindfulness. Establishing boundaries around screen time is an effective way to mitigate these effects, ensuring that technology enhances rather than detracts from our well-being.

To foster mindful technology use, consider setting designated screen-free times throughout your day. These can be moments when you focus on activities that don't involve a screen, such as enjoying a meal with family, taking a walk, or engaging in a hobby. Creating these tech-free zones allows your mind to rest and recharge, reducing the cognitive load that constant screen interaction imposes. Additionally, apps designed to monitor and limit screen usage can be incredibly helpful. They provide insights into your screen time habits, helping you identify patterns and make conscious choices about when and how you use digital devices. By being aware of your screen time, you can take proactive steps to create a more balanced and mindful lifestyle.

Digital detox practices offer a refreshing break from the constant barrage of notifications and updates. Taking regular breaks from screens can significantly enhance your overall well-being. You'll likely notice increased focus and productivity as your mind becomes less cluttered with digital distractions. When you're not constantly switching between apps or web pages, you can concentrate more effectively on the task at hand. Improved sleep quality is another benefit of reducing screen time, especially before bed. The blue light emitted by screens can interfere with your natural sleep-wake cycle, making it harder to fall asleep and stay asleep. By limiting screen exposure in the evening, you create a more conducive environment for restful sleep, leading to better mental and physical health.

Creating a balanced digital lifestyle requires intentionality and commitment. Start by prioritizing offline activities that bring you joy and fulfillment. Whether it's reading a book, gardening, or spending time with loved ones, these activities offer meaningful engagement without the need for screens. Incorporating mindfulness practices into your daily routine can also help you stay grounded and present. This might involve simple breathing exercises, meditation, or just taking a moment to appreciate your surroundings. These practices encourage you to connect with the world around you, fostering a sense of peace and contentment that technology often disrupts. By making space for these moments, you nurture your mental health and cultivate a more balanced approach to technology use.

As you navigate the digital landscape, remember that the goal isn't to eliminate technology from your life but to use it mindfully and purposefully. By finding harmony between screen time and mindful living, you create a sustainable lifestyle that supports your well-being. This balance empowers you to enjoy the benefits of technology without becoming overwhelmed by its demands. With a conscious approach, you can harness the power of digital tools to enhance your life while maintaining a strong connection to the present moment and the world around you.

Chapter 9

Conclusion

As you reach the end of this journey, I hope you've found a friend in these pages, guiding you toward a more balanced and fulfilling lifestyle. We've explored the interconnectedness of mindful nutrition, holistic exercise, and sustainable weight loss, and how these elements work together to create a healthier you. Throughout the book, we've delved into the mind-body connection, emphasizing the importance of integrating mindfulness into your daily routines. This isn't just about counting calories or reps; it's about nurturing your entire self—mind, body, and spirit.

Let's take a moment to revisit the key insights we've uncovered. The benefits of connecting with your body and mind can't be overstated. Mindful eating transforms meals into moments of awareness and pleasure, helping you to savor each bite and understand your body's needs. Creating personalized fitness plans has empowered you to tailor your routines to fit your life, making exercise an enjoyable part of your day rather than a chore. We've tackled stress, revealing ways to manage it effectively through mindfulness and reflection.

The holistic approach we've advocated goes beyond traditional health advice. It's about adopting wellness practices that encourage self-reflection and growth. Through journaling, you've been invited to engage actively with the material, fostering self-awareness and personal development. This practice isn't just a task; it's a journey into understanding yourself better, uncovering what truly drives and fulfills you.

Now, it's time to take these strategies and techniques and weave them into the fabric of your everyday life. Consistency is key. Develop a routine that includes the exercises, meal plans, and mindfulness practices we've discussed. It might be setting aside time for a morning workout, preparing meals mindfully, or practicing deep breathing before bed. Whatever it is, make it yours.

You've been equipped with the tools to transform your life, and I encourage you to embrace this journey with confidence. Imagine the potential that lies ahead—a healthier, more vibrant you. Remember, transformation doesn't happen overnight. It's a gradual process, one that requires patience and persistence. But with each step, you move closer to the life you envision.

As you move forward, I invite you to join online communities and connect with others who share your goals. Share your experiences, learn from others, and find motivation in the stories of those who have walked this path before you. Use technology and apps to track your progress and maintain accountability. These tools can be your allies, helping you stay focused and inspired.

For ongoing support, keep an eye out for additional resources I may offer, be it through a website, app, or social media. These platforms can provide further guidance and updates, ensuring you're never alone in your wellness journey.

Thank you for trusting us and this book to guide you. Your commitment to your health and well-being is inspiring, and I'm confident that you have what it takes to achieve holistic wellness. Embrace this journey with an open heart and mind, knowing that every small step counts.

As you continue on this path, remember this: "The journey of a thousand miles begins with a single step." Live mindfully, cherish each day, and celebrate every victory, no matter how small. Here's to a healthier, happier you.

Extended Edition: Travel-Friendly Workouts

No gym? No problem. These zero-equipment circuits fit in any hotel room, park or small indoor space, keep your momentum on the road. Each circuit takes 8–15 minutes—just you, your bodyweight and common surfaces.

How to use

- Pick one circuit per session either morning, midday or evening

- Aim for 2–3 sessions on travel days; swap circuits to stay engaged

- Move at your own pace—rest 30 seconds between exercises or rounds

1 – Bodyweight Blast (10 minutes)

1. **Air Squats × 15**
   Stand with feet hip-width apart, toes pointing slightly outward. Hinge at the hips and bend your knees, lowering your hips back as if sitting into an invisible chair. Keep your chest lifted and weight in your heels. Drive through your heels to return to standing, squeezing glutes at the top.

2. **Incline Push-ups × 12**
   Place hands shoulder-width on a sturdy surface (bed or desk). Walk your feet back until your body forms a straight line from head to heels. Bend elbows to lower your chest toward the edge, keeping elbows at about 45°. Press through palms to straighten arms, bracing core throughout.

3. **Walking Lunges × 10 steps each leg**
   Step your right foot forward into a deep lunge, dropping your back knee toward the floor. Keep your front knee tracking over your ankle and torso upright. Push through the front heel to stand, then immediately step the left foot forward for the next lunge.

4. **Tricep Dips × 12**
   Sit on the edge of a chair, hands gripping the edge beside your hips. Slide your butt off the chair, legs ex-

tended in front. Lower your body by bending elbows until they reach about 90°, keeping shoulders down. Press through palms to straighten arms, engaging triceps.

5. **Mountain Climbers × 30 seconds**
Start in a high plank with hands beneath shoulders. Drive your right knee toward your chest, then quickly switch legs in a running motion. Keep hips steady and core tight—avoid sagging or piking.

Repeat 2 rounds

2 – Park Circuit (12 minutes)

1. **Bench Step-ups × 12 each leg**
Stand facing a bench or low wall. Place your right foot on the bench, press through your heel, and lift your body until your right leg is straight. Lower back slowly and switch legs.

2. **Push-ups on Bench × 10**
Hands on bench, feet on ground, body in straight line. Bend elbows to lower chest toward bench, keeping core braced. Press through palms to return.

1. **Bulgarian Split Squats × 10 each leg**
   Stand a couple of feet in front of the bench, place your rear foot on the bench's edge. Lower your front thigh until it's parallel to the ground, keeping front knee over ankle. Press through front heel to rise.

2. **Bench Plank × 30 seconds**
   Forearms on bench, feet on ground, body in a straight line. Squeeze glutes, draw belly button to spine, and hold without letting hips sag.

3. **Bench Jump-overs × 20 total**
   Stand to one side of bench. Bend knees, jump sideways over bench, landing softly on the balls of your feet with knees slightly bent. Repeat back.

Repeat 2 rounds

3 – Core & Balance Flow (8 minutes)

1. **Plank Shoulder Taps × 20 (10 per shoulder)**
   In high plank, feet wider than hip-width. Keeping hips stable, lift one hand to tap the opposite shoulder. Alternate sides, minimizing torso rotation.

2. **Single-Leg Deadlifts × 10 each leg**
   Stand tall, shift weight onto right foot. Hinge at hips, extend left leg straight back and reach hands toward

the floor. Keep back flat and shoulders square. Return to start and switch sides.

3. **Side Plank (Right) × 30 seconds**
   Lie on right side, forearm under shoulder, legs stacked. Lift hips until body forms a straight line. Hold, then switch sides.

4. **Side Plank (Left) × 30 seconds**
   Same form on your left side.

5. **Bird-Dog × 12 each side**
   On hands and knees, extend right arm forward and left leg back simultaneously. Keep hips level. Return and repeat with opposite limbs.

Perform as a straight set

4 – Stairs & Step Burn (15 minutes)

1. **Stair Run × 5 rounds**
   Sprint up a flight of stairs, using arms to drive. Walk back down for recovery.

2. **Calf Raises × 20**
   Stand on bottom stair edge, heels hanging off. Rise onto toes, pause, then lower until heels dip below step level.

3. **Incline Push-ups on Step × 12**

   Hands on bottom step, feet on ground. Keep body straight, lower chest to step, then press up.

4. **Decline Plank × 30 seconds**

   Feet on bottom step, hands on floor. Keep body rigid and core braced.

5. **Step Jump-ups × 10**

   Stand facing step. Bend knees, swing arms, and jump both feet onto step. Step down one foot at a time.

Repeat 2 rounds

5 – Express Upper-Body Pump (8 minutes)

1. **Push-ups × 12**

   Hands shoulder-width, body in straight line. Lower chest until elbows reach 90°, then press up.

2. **Chair Dips × 12**

   Hands on chair behind you, fingers facing forward. Lower hips until elbows bend 90°, then press up.

3. **Pike Push-ups × 10**

   From a "V" shape (hips high), bend elbows to lower head toward floor. Press back up, focusing on shoulder engagement.

4. **Reverse Plank × 30 seconds**

   Sit with legs extended, hands behind hips. Lift hips until body forms a straight line from head to heels.

5. **Arm Circles × 30 seconds each direction**

   Stand tall, arms out to sides. Make small circles forward for 30 seconds, then backward for 30 seconds.

Perform as a straight set

Sample Travel Day Plan

Morning – Wake-Up Charge
  – Bodyweight Blast (10 minutes)

Midday – Desk Detox
  – Core & Balance Flow (8 minutes)

Evening – Pre-Sleep Reset
  – Express Upper-Body Pump (8 minutes) + gentle full-body stretch (5 minutes)

Bonus Chapter: Fitness Myths Debunked

Separating Fact from Fiction

The world of fitness is full of information — some of it incredibly helpful, and some of it downright misleading. In this bonus chapter, we'll tackle some of the most common fitness myths and uncover the truths behind them to help you approach your fitness journey with confidence and clarity.

Introduction to the Bonus Chapter

Congratulations on reaching the conclusion of this book! As a special addition, this bonus chapter is designed to clear up common misconceptions that can hold you back or cause unnecessary confusion on your path to wellness. Let's get started on separating fact from fiction in the world of fitness.

Myth 1: Cardio is the Best Way to Lose Weight

The Truth: While cardio exercises like running and cycling are excellent for burning calories, they're not the only path to weight loss. Resistance training is equally important because it helps build muscle, which boosts your metabolism and leads to more calories burned even at rest. The best approach is a combination of both cardio and strength training for sustainable results.

Myth 2: Lifting Weights Makes Women Bulky

The Truth: This myth persists despite overwhelming evidence to the contrary. Women typically don't produce enough testosterone to gain massive muscle mass like men. Lifting weights can help women achieve a toned and sculpted physique, improve bone density, and enhance overall strength.

Myth 3: No Pain, No Gain

The Truth: While pushing yourself during workouts is important, pain is not a requirement for progress. Discomfort can signal effort, but sharp or persistent pain is your body's way of warning you about potential injury. Listen to your body and prioritize proper form and recovery to prevent setbacks.

Myth 4: You Can Target Fat Loss in Specific Areas

The Truth: Spot reduction, or targeting fat loss in specific areas through exercises, is a myth. When you lose fat, it happens across your entire body, not just the areas you work on. Consistent exercise, paired with a balanced diet, is the key to overall fat loss.

Myth 5: More Workouts Mean Faster Results

The Truth: Overtraining can actually hinder your progress and increase your risk of injury. Rest and recovery are essential components of any fitness routine. Muscles need time to repair and grow stronger, so incorporate rest days and prioritize sleep.

Myth 6: Stretching Before a Workout Prevents Injuries

The Truth: While stretching is important, static stretching (holding a stretch for a prolonged time) before a workout might not be the best choice. Dynamic warm-ups, which involve active movements that mimic your workout, are more effective in preparing your body and reducing the risk of injury.

Myth 7: You Need to Work Out Every Day to See Results

The Truth: Consistency is crucial, but quality matters more than quantity. A well-structured fitness routine with 3-5 days of focused exercise, complemented by active recovery and rest, can yield excellent results. Overworking yourself can lead to burnout and diminishing returns.

Myth 8: Crunches are the Best Way to Get Abs

The Truth: Crunches alone won't give you a six-pack. A strong core requires a mix of exercises that target different abdominal muscles, along with a healthy diet to reduce body fat. Planks, leg raises, and rotational movements are excellent additions to your core routine.

Myth 9: Eating More Protein Will Automatically Build Muscle

The Truth: Protein is vital for muscle repair and growth, but simply eating more protein without engaging in strength training won't lead to muscle gain. Pair your protein intake with resistance exercises to achieve optimal results.

Myth 10: Sweating More Means a Better Workout

The Truth: Sweating is your body's way of cooling down, not a measure of workout intensity or calorie burn. Factors like temperature, humidity, and individual differences influence how much you sweat. Focus on effort and proper technique rather than how much you sweat.

Myth 11: Fitness Requires Expensive Gym Memberships or Equipment

The Truth: You don't need a gym membership or fancy equipment to stay fit. Bodyweight exercises, outdoor activities, and affordable equipment like resistance bands can provide an effective workout. Fitness is about creativity and consistency, not cost.

Myth 12: Morning Workouts Are Better Than Evening Workouts

The Truth: The best time to work out is whenever you feel most energetic and can maintain consistency. Both morning and evening workouts have their advantages, so choose a time that aligns with your schedule and preferences.

Myth 13: Older Adults Should Avoid Strength Training

The Truth: Strength training is beneficial for people of all ages, including older adults. It helps maintain muscle mass, improve bone density, and enhance overall functionality, reducing the risk of falls and injuries.

Myth 14: If You're Not Sore, You Didn't Work Hard Enough

The Truth: Muscle soreness is not an accurate indicator of workout effectiveness. While some soreness is normal when trying new exercises, consistent training improves your recovery. Focus on progress in strength, endurance, and mobility instead.

Myth 15: Supplements Are Necessary for Fitness Success

The Truth: While some supplements can be helpful, they're not essential for achieving fitness goals. A balanced diet rich in whole foods can provide most of the nutrients you need. Consult a healthcare professional before adding supplements to your routine.

Final Thoughts

By dispelling these myths, you can approach fitness with a clearer understanding of what works and what doesn't. Remember, there's no one-size-fits-all approach to fitness. Listen to your body, embrace a balanced routine, and focus on long-term health rather than quick fixes.

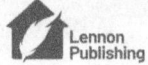

Thank you for reading *The Ultimate Holistic Essentials: A Complete Wellness and Fitness Collection with Mindfulness and Healthy Diet for Everyday Living.*

If this collection helped you build better habits, feel more balanced, or inspired new routines, we'd truly appreciate your feedback. Your review helps more readers discover practical ways to bring mindfulness and fitness into their daily lives.

You can scan the QR code or visit our review page to share your thoughts. It only takes a moment but makes a lasting difference for independent publishers like us.

References

- Anderida Practice. (n.d.). *The holistic benefits of exercise for health and wellbeing*. Retrieved from https://www.theanderidapractice.com/news-all-posts/the-holistic-benefits-of-exercise-for-health-and-wellbeing

- Boss As A Service. (n.d.). *Using a workout accountability app to stick to your fitness plan*. Retrieved from https://bossasaservice.com/blog/workout-accountability-app/

- Business Insider. (n.d.). *Best mood trackers for mental health management*. Retrieved from https://www.businessinsider.com/guides/health/mental-health/mood-tracker

- Clear, J. (n.d.). *How to build new habits by taking advantage of old ones*. Retrieved from https://jamesclear.com/habit-stacking

- Clear, J. (n.d.). *How to master the art of continuous im-

provement. Retrieved from https://jamesclear.com/continuous-improvement

- Clear, J. (n.d.). *How to stick with good habits even when your willpower is low*. Retrieved from https://jamesclear.com/choice-architecture

- DFDRussell. (n.d.). *Digital detox: Managing screen time for better mental health*. Retrieved from https://www.dfdrussell.org/digital-detox-managing-screen-time-for-better-mental-health/

- EVŌLVE Strong. (n.d.). *Personalized fitness plans for better health*. Retrieved from https://evolvstrong.com/the-science-behind-custom-fitness-plans-why-personalization-leads-to-better-health-outcomes/

- Fitness CF Gyms. (n.d.). *Time-efficient workouts for busy lifestyles*. Retrieved from https://fitnesscfgyms.com/mountdorafl/blog/fitness-tips/time-efficient-workouts-for-busy-lifestyles/

- Graybiel, A. M. (2008). The basal ganglia and habit formation. Nature Reviews Neuroscience, 7(6), 464–476. https://doi.org/10.1038/nrn1919

- Harvard T.H. Chan School of Public Health. (n.d.). *Healthy eating plate*. Retrieved from https://nutrition

source.hsph.harvard.edu/healthy-eating-plate/

- Healthline. (n.d.). *Mindful eating 101 — A beginner's guide*. Retrieved from https://www.healthline.com/nutrition/mindful-eating-guide

- Healthline. (n.d.). *The 8 best calorie counter apps*. Retrieved from https://www.healthline.com/nutrition/best-calorie-counters

- HumanGood. (n.d.). *7 low-impact exercises for older adults to stay active*. Retrieved from https://www.humangood.org/resources/senior-living-blog/low-impact-exercises-for-older-adults

- Johns Hopkins Medicine. (n.d.). *Hunger and fullness awareness*. Retrieved from https://www.hopkinsmedicine.org/health/wellness-and-prevention/hunger-and-fullness-awareness

- Mayo Clinic. (n.d.). *Mindfulness exercises*. Retrieved from https://www.mayoclinic.org/healthy-lifestyle/consumer-health/in-depth/mindfulness-exercises/art-20046356

- Mayo Clinic. (n.d.). *Positive thinking: Stop negative self-talk to reduce stress*. Retrieved from https://www.mayoclinic.org/healthy-lifestyle/stress

-management/in-depth/positive-thinking/art-20043950

- Mindful Leader. (n.d.). *7 breathing exercises for a balanced mind and body*. Retrieved from https://www.mindfulleader.org/blog/88637-harnessing-the-power-of-breath-7

- MindTools. (n.d.). *Visualization – Imagining and achieving your goals*. Retrieved from https://www.mindtools.com/a5ycdws/visualization

- National Center for Biotechnology Information. (2021). *Web workouts and consumer well-being: The role of digital fitness programs*. Retrieved from https://pmc.ncbi.nlm.nih.gov/articles/PMC8242656/

- National Center for Biotechnology Information. (2024). *Effects of mindfulness-based interventions on promoting mental health and well-being*. Retrieved from https://pmc.ncbi.nlm.nih.gov/articles/PMC9915077/#:~:text=In%20a%20Swiss%20study%20%5B33,helping%20them%20to%20perform%20better.

- Natural Resources Defense Council. (n.d.). *Industrial agricultural pollution 101*. Retrieved from https://www.nrdc.org/stories/industrial-agricul

tural-pollution-101

- Nutrition by Kristin. (n.d.). *100+ intuitive and mindful eating journal prompts from an intuitive eating dietitian*. Retrieved from https://nutritionbykristin.com/intuitive-and-mindful-eating-journal-prompts-from-an-intuitive-eating-dietitian/

- One Tree Planted. (n.d.). *9 tips for sustainable eating*. Retrieved from https://onetreeplanted.org/blogs/stories/9-tips-sustainable-eating

- Planet Forward. (n.d.). *Research shows plant-based diets better for your health*. Retrieved from https://planetforward.org/story/plant-based-diets-health/

- Positive Psychology. (n.d.). *5 benefits of journaling for mental health*. Retrieved from https://positivepsychology.com/benefits-of-journaling/#:~:text=Research%20suggests%20that%20expressive%20writing,lasting%20longer%20than%2030%20days.

- Tastewise. (n.d.). *Sustainable food sourcing: Data-driven strategies*. Retrieved from https://tastewise.io/blog/sustainable-food-sourcing#:~:text=Sustainable%20food%20sourcing%20is%20t he,local%20and%20small%2Dscale%20producers.

- United States Environmental Protection Agency. (n.d.). *Preventing wasted food at home.* Retrieved from https://www.epa.gov/recycle/preventing-wasted-food-home

- Verywell Mind. (n.d.). *Body scan meditation: Benefits and how to do it.* Retrieved from https://www.verywellmind.com/body-scan-meditation-why-and-how-3144782

- Wirecutter. (2025). *The 4 best meditation apps of 2025.* Retrieved from https://www.nytimes.com/wirecutter/reviews/best-meditation-apps/

www.ingramcontent.com/pod-product-compliance
Lightning Source LLC
Chambersburg PA
CBHW020531030426
42337CB00013B/801